International Research on Poverty Reduction

This book series covers poverty reduction practices and experience, knowledge mobilization, poverty reduction strategy analysis, and comparative research of different poverty reduction models. By analyzing China's poverty reduction approaches and experiences, and comparing them with those of other countries, this book series provides policy makers, researchers and practitioners in poverty reduction with theoretical and technical support, as well asproviding a new channel for sharing experiences as well as facilitating collaboration and communication in poverty reduction development fields between China and the rest of the world. Poverty remains a crucial development issue for the world, and China has become an important player in the global endeavor in poverty reduction and development. China has made a substantial contribution to the achievement of the Millennium Development Goals (MDGs) by reducing half of its poverty population.

More information about this series at http://www.springer.com/series/11685

Xiaolin Wang · Xiaoying Zhang

Towards 2030 – China's Poverty Alleviation and Global Poverty Governance

SSAP

Springer

Xiaolin Wang
The Institute for Six-sector Economy
Fudan University
Shanghai, China

Xiaoying Zhang
The Institute for Six-sector Economy
Fudan University
Shanghai, China

Translated by
Xiaoling Yue
Global Tone Communication
Technology Co., Ltd.
Beijing, China

Lin Jingxian
Global Tone Communication
Technology Co., Ltd.
Beijing, China

Sponsored by the Chinese Fund for the Humanities and Social Sciences

ISSN 2195-9781 ISSN 2195-979X (electronic)
International Research on Poverty Reduction
ISBN 978-981-15-6355-3 ISBN 978-981-15-6356-0 (eBook)
https://doi.org/10.1007/978-981-15-6356-0

Jointly published with Social Sciences Academic Press
The print edition is not for sale in China (Mainland). Customers from China (Mainland) please order the print book from: Social Sciences Academic Press.

This Springer imprint is published by the registered company Springer Nature Singapore Pte Ltd.
The registered company address is: 152 Beach Road, #21-01/04 Gateway East, Singapore 189721, Singapore

Contents

Chapter 1
China's Success in Poverty Reduction and Its Contribution to Worldwide Progress Toward MDGs

China's remarkable achievements in poverty reduction in recent years have made it the first developing country to achieve the poverty-reduction target set by the Millennium Development Goals (MDGs). On its journey toward eradicating poverty, China has explored a few models befitting its national conditions. Apart from a focus on both government-led development programs and the social security system, the country gives full play to the roles of market and the general public in poverty reduction. In the meanwhile, China has taken an active part in improving global poverty governance. It strengthens international exchanges and cooperation in this area, sharing its good practices with other developing countries to help them achieve the MDGs and Sustainable Development Goals (SDGs) of the United Nations. This chapter begins with an overview of the progress toward MDGs' poverty-reduction targets before examining China's progress toward the targets and the country's contributions to the global fight against poverty.

1.1 MDG Poverty-Reduction Targets: Background, Action Plans and Achievements

1.1.1 Launch of the Targets

The year 2000 marks a milestone in the history of international development. At the United Nations Millennium Summit held in September of that year, leaders of 189 countries signed *the United Nations Millennium Declaration* (hereinafter referred to as the "Millennium Declaration"). The Declaration was translated into a roadmap setting out specific goals and targets to be reached by 2015, called the Millennium Development Goals (MDGs), incorporating eight goals of halving the proportion of

X. Wang and X. Zhang, *Towards 2030 – China's Poverty Alleviation and Global Poverty Governance*, International Research on Poverty Reduction,
https://doi.org/10.1007/978-981-15-6356-0_1

Table 1.1 MDGs' goal 1: Eradicate extreme poverty and hunger

Serial number	Contents
Target 1.A	Halve, between 1990 and 2015, the proportion of people whose income is less than one dollar a day
Target 1.B	Achieve full and productive employment and decent work for all, including women and young people
Target 1.C	Halve, between 1990 and 2015, the proportion of people who suffer from hunger

Source Resolution 55/162 adopted by the UN general assembly

poverty-stricken people between 1990 and 2015, achieving universal primary education, promoting gender equality, reducing maternal and child mortality, combating HIV/AIDS and malaria, ensuring environmental sustainability, and developing a global partnership for development.

To help track and measure progress toward these eight goals, 21 targets and 60 indicators were developed. The primary goal of MDGs is to "eradicate extreme poverty and hunger," comprising the following three targets. Target 1.A is to halve, between 1990 and 2015, the proportion of people whose income is less than one dollar a day, and the poverty line was later raised to USD 1.25 at 2005 purchasing power parity (PPP).[1] Target 1.B is to achieve full and productive employment and decent work for all, including women and young people. Target 1.C is to halve, between 1990 and 2015, the proportion of people who suffer from hunger. We believe that targets 1.A and 1.C constitute the goal of eradicating extreme poverty and hunger, while target 1.C is an important means of achieving them (see Table 1.1).

Between 1981 and 1990, roughly 1,950 million people lived in extreme poverty across the world. In the following decade until 2000, the number dropped from 1,926 million to 1,700 million, with a slight decrease of 226 million. But it was not the case in sub-Saharan Africa where the scale and proportion of poor population increased instead, or in South Asia where extreme poverty remained a major challenge. In this context, the United Nations Millennium Summit in 2000 made it one of the biggest global challenges to "eradicate extreme poverty." The target to "halve the proportion of poor people" is a world-recognized development indicator that receives the most extensive, comprehensive and specific support.[2]

Poverty reduction has been made the overriding goal of MDGs not only because poverty poses the biggest obstacle for socioeconomic development of developing countries, but more importantly, poverty reduction is at the heart of all goals. The failure to achieve Goal 1 would make it impossible to attain Goal 2–7. Even if temporary relief could be achieved through short-term assistance programs, the results cannot be sustained.

---

[1]The poverty line was updated to USD 1.25 a day measured at 2005 international prices adjusted for purchasing power parity (PPP).

[2]UN (2005).

1.1.2 Global Actions Toward Poverty Reduction

To achieve the MDGs in all respects, especially the goal of poverty reduction by the scheduled 2015, the signatory countries have jointly pledged to "create an environment—at the national and global levels alike—which is conducive to development and the elimination of poverty," introduce policies and arouse wide public concern over development. Only in this way can it be possible to halve the proportion of over 1.9 billion people in extreme poverty by 2015. Such a "conducive environment" depends on the joint efforts of both developed and developing countries. The developed countries need to increase assistance to developing countries, particularly to Africa, helping removing capital, technological and management obstacles in the backward regions, and enabling the people below the poverty line to achieve leapfrog development. The developing countries have more to do, such as opening up their markets, adopting advanced development ideas, and expanding and deepening new-type South–South cooperation.

In accordance with the *United Nations Millennium Declaration* and the *Road Map towards the Implementation of the United Nations Millennium Declaration* (hereinafter referred to as the Road Map), the implementing bodies of MDGs constitute three groups: UN and other international development agencies, developed countries (mainly OECD-DAC member countries) and developing countries. The participants include signatory governments, the UN system, intergovernmental organizations, international and regional agencies, among others.[3]

1. Role and actions of the United Nations

The Millennium Declaration, the Road Map and various initiatives have all mentioned to enhance the role of the UN in achieving the MDGs, mainly in top-level planning, policy dialogue, demonstration projects and accountability supervision. Apart from the above-mentioned Road Map, the UN has led various types of planning and feasibility studies, such as the UN Millennium Project between 2002 and 2005. Led by the United Nations Development Programme (UNDP), the project was carried out by 10 task forces comprising more than 250 experts. Based on the survey into seven countries, including Dominican Republic and Ethiopia, the project analyzed the progress and difficulties during the implementation of MDGs and developed a feasible global action plan to fulfill the commitments of MDGs by 2015. The project report, consisting of one master report and 13 sub-reports, released in 2005 with a master report and 13 sub-reports, is recognized by the UN as comprehensive.[4]

To meet the poor countries' need for external aids, the UN has promoted North-South cooperation through effective and genuine dialogues among development organizations, countries, as well as a raft of preferential policies. Such efforts include the WTO Doha round of multilateral trade negotiations in 2001, UN General Assembly Special Session on HIV/AIDS in 2001, *Brussels Programme of Action for the Least*

[3]UN (2001).

[4]UN Millennium Project (2005).

Developed Countries adopted in 2001, International Conference on Financing for Development in 2002, the 2005 World Summit and *The Paris Declaration on Aid Effectiveness* adopted in 2005.[5]

In addition, the UN carried out demonstration projects for rural development, such as the Millennium Villages Project (MVP) jointly developed by the UNDP, Japanese government and Columbia University. Instead of setting up new villages, the MVP chose existing African villages with relative political stability but in severe poverty and hunger, with a view to improving the living conditions of the poor through agricultural development. Between 2004 and 2006, the MVP was carried out in 12 villages located in Ethiopia, Ghana, Kenya, Malawi, Mali, Nigeria, Rwanda, Senegal, Tanzania and Uganda.

The UN played an important role in monitoring and evaluation as well. Following a raft of policies and actions toward MDGs, it mobilized the private sector, non-government agencies and other social forces by various means to actively participate in and monitor the MDGs projects. It also developed a meticulous self-monitoring and third-party evaluation system. In accordance with the UN Resolution 55/162 adopted on December 18, 2000 and the UN Resolution 56/95 adopted on December 14, 2001, the Secretary-General of the UN is requested to prepare an annual report on progress achieved by the United Nations system and member states in implementing the Millennium Declaration. In 2005, the Inter-Agency and Expert Group on MDG Indicators began to publicly release The Millennium Development Goals Report on a yearly basis. The Group is led by the Department of Economic and Social Affairs of the United Nations Secretariat, comprising representatives from a number of UN agencies, such as United Nations Environment Programme (UNEP) and UNDP, as well as from international organizations outside the UN system, like the World Bank and IMF.

2. Role and actions of developed countries

MDGs indicate that the poverty and inequality across the world could be fundamentally attributed to many developing countries, especially those in Africa, that have been marginalized in the process of globalization. During the global economic boom in the 1990s, these poor countries benefited little from world trade, investment and technological progress. Given their lack in factors and home-grown driving force for development, the extensive global intervention has been made a must for the development of these countries and for the delivery of benefits from economic development to the least developed regions.

Such global intervention is mainly achieved by increasing the official development assistance (ODA) from developed countries, referring to the member states of the Organization for Economic Cooperation and Development's Development Assistance Committee (OECD-DAC). The MDGs roadmap calls for increasing international development assistance for multiple times and setting out the "Goal 8" to help track progress toward the developed countries' commitment "to take special

[5]OECD (2005).

measures to address the challenges of poverty eradication and sustainable development in Africa, including debt cancellation, improved market access, enhanced ODA and increased flows of foreign direct investment, as well as drugs and technology." Specifically, it includes the commitment by DAC member states to contribute 0.7% of their gross national income (GNI) as ODA, double aid to Africa, increase aid to the least developed countries (LDCs), increase aid for trade to developing countries, expand the developing countries' duty-free access to the markets of developed countries, among others. Judging from the annual reports on MDGs, however, the commitment has never been fulfilled, especially after the financial crisis.

Take ODA for instance. According to the Millennium Declaration, *Brussels Programme of Action for the Least Developed Countries for the Decade 2001–2010* and the *2002 Monterrey Consensus of the International Conference on Financing for Development*, DAC member states should contribute 0.7% of their GNI as ODA to developing countries. From 2000 to 2015, Luxembourg, Denmark, Norway and Sweden were the only countries that did so every year, the Netherlands and the UK met the target for some years, while some traditional donors, like the USA, never met the target. The average ODA/GNI of the DAC member states stood at 0.2–0.3% (see Fig. 1.1).

3. Missions and actions of developing countries

Among the MDGs signatories, a large number of developing countries, especially those in Africa, are the most marginalized in the process of globalization. Apart from a favorable external environment, efforts from within these countries are needed if

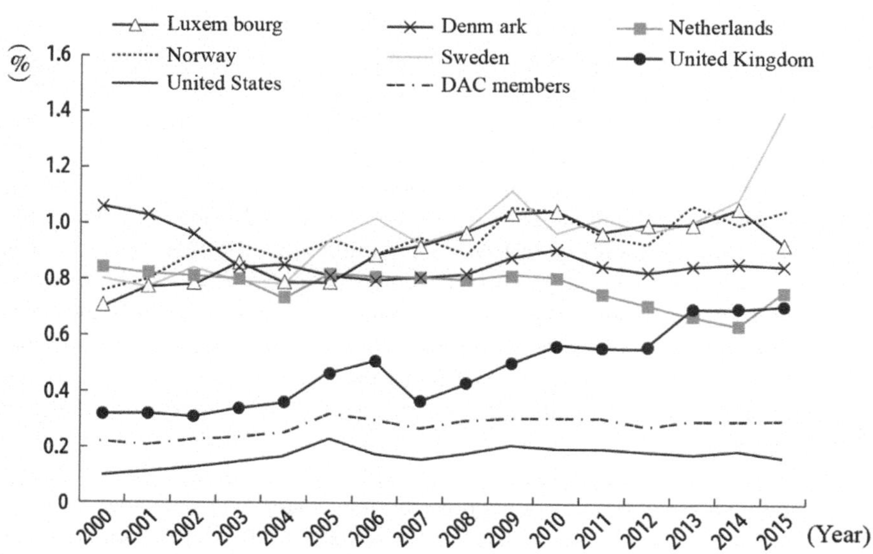

Fig. 1.1 ODA/GNI of DAC members and some other countries (2000–2015). *Source* https://data.oecd.org/oda/net-oda.htm

they are to achieve MDGs. Unlike Agenda 21, another global action plan of the UN, the MDGs signatories are not required to develop corresponding national roadmaps to ensure the attainment of the goals. Driven by the awareness-raising efforts of the United Nations, African leaders have pledged on various occasions to make sure governments uphold the rule of law, human rights, democracy, good governance, and open markets, strengthen infrastructure, support agriculture and manufacturing, boost education, training and services, and step up efforts to prevent HIV/AIDS and other infectious diseases. However, most developing countries would incorporate MDGs into their national mid- and long-term development strategies and policies, instead of putting together a policy package designed specifically for MDGs. In Africa, in particular, the lack of funds has become the root cause for the failure of many policies.

The UN has observed in the early-stage assessment that Africa would be a key area for poverty production: about half of its population on the continent lives below the poverty line.[6] That was why UN has since the very beginning adopted action plans geared toward meeting the special needs of Africa. These include efforts to build a new type of partnership with African countries and to establish the African Union. Other than that, however, the UN imposed no requirements on each country in terms of actions to be taken.

1.1.3 Progress of MDGs in Poverty Reduction

Thanks to the joint efforts of the UN and various actors over the first 15 years since the launch of MDGs in 2000, the targets of "halving the proportion of people living below the poverty line and of people who suffer from hunger" have been reached, despite the impact of global disasters like the 2008 financial crisis and some regional security issues. To begin with, as we reach the end of the MDG period, extreme poverty has declined significantly. In 1990, nearly half of the population in the developing world lived on less than USD 1.25 a day; that proportion dropped to 14% in 2015. Second, the number of people living in extreme poverty has declined globally by more than half, falling from 1,926 million in 1990 to 836 million in 2015. Most progress has occurred since 2000 (see Fig. 1.2). Third, the number of people in the working middle class—living on more than USD 4 a day—has almost tripled between 1991 and 2015. This group now makes up half the workforce in the developing regions, up from just 18% in 1991. Fourth, the proportion of undernourished people in the developing regions has fallen by almost half since 1990, from 23.3% in 1990–1992 to 12.9% in 2014–2016.[7]

Results differed among different regions, with Asia consistently outperforming Africa, and East and Southeast Asia outperforming South Asia. The goal of eradicating extreme poverty and hunger has been achieved overall, but to various degrees

---

[6]UN (2002).

[7]UN (2015).

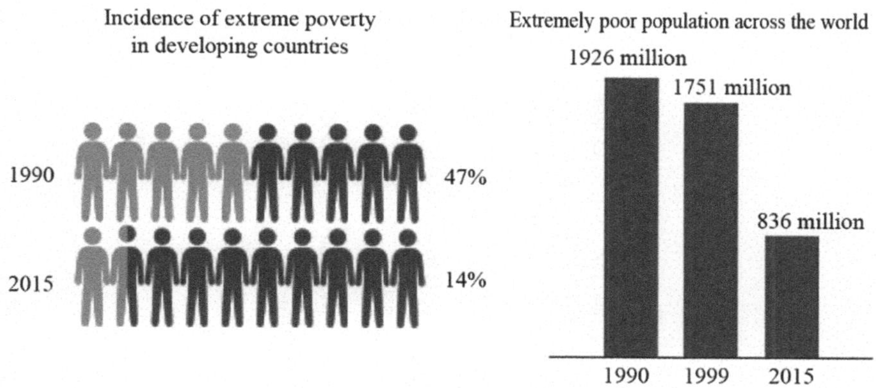

Fig. 1.2 Goal 1: Eradicate extreme poverty and hunger. *Source* The Millennium Development Goals Report (2015)

across regions. The proportions of the people living below the poverty line and the people who suffer from hunger are still extremely high in sub-Saharan Africa and South Asia (see Table 1.2).

Despite enormous progress, even today, about 800 million people still live in extreme poverty and suffer from hunger. Over 160 million children under age five have inadequate height for their age due to insufficient food. Currently, 57 million children of primary school age are not in school. Almost half of global workers are still working in vulnerable conditions, with little access to the benefits that come with decent work.

1.2 China's Progress Toward MDGs in Poverty Reduction

1.2.1 The Poor Population Dropped Significantly and the Basic Needs of Rural Residents have been Basically Met

Boasting tremendous achievements in poverty reduction, China has become the first country to achieve the MDGs in poverty reduction. Measured against the international poverty line of USD 1.25 a day (2005 PPP), the incidence of poverty dropped from 74% in 1990 to 4% in 2005. China had reduced the number of people living in extreme poverty by over 700 million since 1981 (see Fig. 1.3). The targets of "halving the proportion of people living below the poverty line" and "halving the proportion of people who suffer from hunger" under the Goal 1 of MDGs have been over-fulfilled (see Table 1.3).

China's remarkable progress in poverty reduction has contributed enormously to the global poverty reduction. It brought the proportion of people living in extreme

Table 1.2 Progress of MDGs in poverty reduction (2015)

Targets	Africa		Asia				Oceania	Latin America and the Caribbean	Caucasus and Central Asia
	Northern	Sub-Saharan	Easton	Southeastern	Southern	Western			
Reduce extreme poverty by half	Low poverty	Very high poverty	Low poverty	Moderate poverty	High poverty	Low poverty	–	Low poverty	Low poverty
Productive and decent employment	Large deficit	Very large deficit	Moderate deficit	Large deficit	Large deficit	Large deficit	Very large deficit	Moderate deficit	Small deficit
Reduce hunger by half	Low hunger	High hunger	Moderate hunger	Moderate hunger	High hunger	Moderate hunger	Moderate hunger	Moderate hunger	Moderate hunger

Source Millennium development goals: 2015 progress chart, http://www.un.org

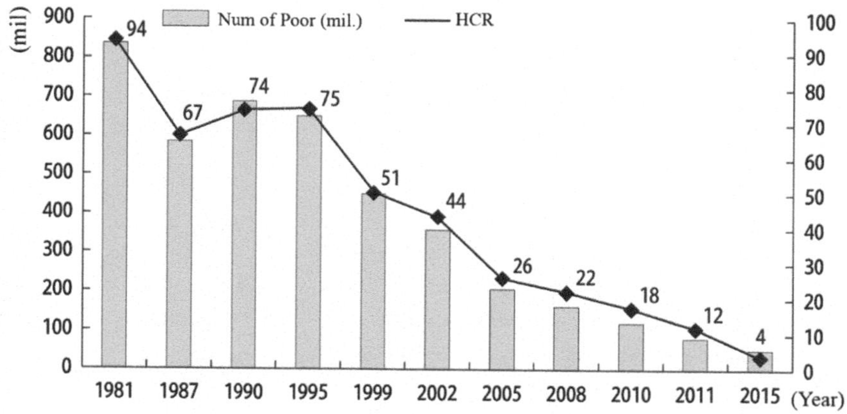

Fig. 1.3 China's poverty reduction and HCR. *Note* Num of Poor (mil) is the number of poor people (unit: million); HCR refers to the head count ratio

Table 1.3 China's progress toward MDGs

Goals and targets	Status
Goal 1: Eradicate extreme poverty and hunger	
Target 1A: Halve, between 1990 and 2015, the proportion of people whose income is less than USD 1.25 a day	Achieved
Target 1B: Achieve full and productive employment and decent work for all, including women and young people	Basically achieved
Target 1C: Halve, between 1990 and 2015, the proportion of people who suffer from hunger	Achieved

Source Ministry of Foreign Affairs of People's Republic of China and United Nations in China: Report on China's Implementation of the Millennium Development Goals (2000–2015), 2015

poverty in East Asia down from 61% in 1990 to 4% in 2015, the most notable decline among all regions of the world. The extreme poverty rate in the developing countries (excluding China) fell by 57% from 41% in 1990 to 18% in 2015, as against a drop of 69% from 47% in 1990 to 14% in 2015 in the developing countries (including China). These numbers demonstrate China's role in reducing global poverty.[8]

China is the most populous developing country in the world. Over the 15 years between 2000 and 2015, China made sustained efforts to strengthen its overall agricultural production capacity. The national output of grain and other agricultural and sideline products continued to grow. In particular, the grain output climbed steadily for 11 consecutive years since 2004, with the grain per capita up to 445 kg in 2014.[9] According to the 2015 Global Hunger Index (GHI) of International Food Policy Research Institute, China saw a decline in GHI from 25.1% in 1990 to 8.6% in 2015,

[8]Huang (2016).

[9]Ministry of Foreign Affairs of People's Republic of China and United Nations in China (2015).

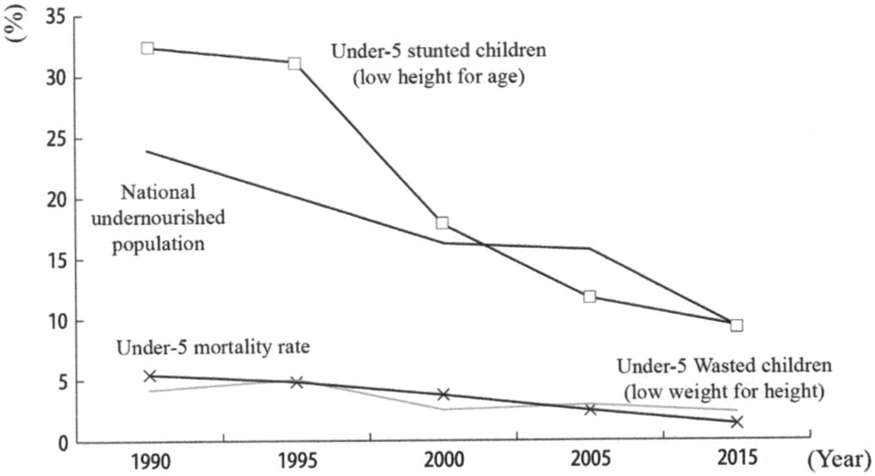

Fig. 1.4 Nutrition in China. *Source* Author's calculations using statistics from the 2015 Global Hunger Index

together with a significant decrease in the proportion of the undernourished population, that of children under age five who suffer from wasting (low weight for height), that of children under age five who suffer from stunting (low height for age) and that of children who die before age five (see Fig. 1.4).[10]

1.2.2 Increasing Income of the Poor Population, Thanks to Various Anti-poverty Policies

China's progress in poverty reduction has been a result of the synergy among various policies. The increasing income in the poverty-stricken areas and the national special poverty-reduction policies are key contributors to the declining incidence of poverty in China, while the increase in the personal income would be impossible without the macroeconomic growth. Since the launch of reform and opening up in 1978, China has carried out policy reforms in land, finance, investment, trade, population and social management, taken advantage of international development assistance, attracted foreign direct investment and expanded international trade. The troika of China's economic growth (investment, consumption and trade) has boosted the steady and rapid growth of the national economy. China's GDP surged from RMB 10 trillion in 2000 to 67.8 trillion in 2015, the second highest in the world, which has been followed by the increase in urban and rural personal income. In 2015 the disposable income of urban residents and the per capita net income of rural residents reached RMB 31,195 and RMB 10,772, respectively (see Fig. 1.5), equaling to 3.6 times and

[10]IFPRI (2015).

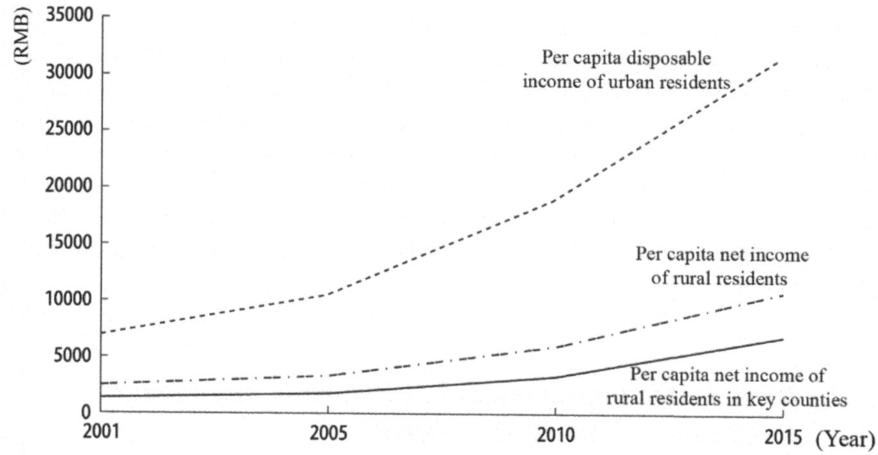

Fig. 1.5 Income of Chinese residents (2001–2015). *Source* National Bureau of statistics: Main survey results of poverty monitoring in Rural China 2015

3.1 times of that in 2000 at comparable prices. Between 2001 and 2015, in national key counties for development-oriented poverty reduction,[11] the average annual growth rate of the per capita net income of farmers and the per capita local GDP surpassed the national average.

Department of Household Surveys of National Bureau of Statistics: Main Data of Household Survey in China 2016.

Special development-oriented poverty-reduction programs targeting poverty-stricken areas and people constitute another important means for China's success in poverty reduction.[12] With a view to improving the production and living conditions in the impoverished areas, China set up the State Council Leading Group of Poverty Alleviation and Development to coordinate the poverty reduction work of all departments and social organizations involved. In addition, the State Council Leading Group Office of Poverty Alleviation and Development was established to function as a national institution dedicated to development-oriented poverty reduction. Moreover, there are dedicated trans-departmental agencies for poverty reduction, tasked to set the poverty line, identify the people living below the poverty line, and set up special funds to support the impoverished areas and the poor people. China has continued to increase the special funds for poverty reduction and carried out *The Seven-Year Program for Lifting 80 Million People out of Poverty (1994–2000), the Outline for Development-Oriented Poverty Reduction for China's Rural*

[11]There is a total of 592 such counties which are the most impoverished and determined according to their performance in such indicators as per capita GDP, per capita disposable financial resources and per capita net income of farmers. They are entitled to national priority support.

[12]The poverty-stricken areas incorporate 832 counties, including those in the contiguous impoverished areas and the key counties for national poverty reduction and development program outside the contiguous impoverished areas. There are 680 counties in the contiguous impoverished areas, containing 440 out of the 562 national key counties for poverty reduction and development.

Areas (2001–2010) and the Outline for Development-Oriented Poverty Reduction for China's Rural Areas (2011–2020), among other national poverty-reduction plans. At different stages of development, appropriate poverty-reduction policies relating to infrastructure construction, public services, industrial growth, small-loan guarantee program, ecological compensation and others are introduced. Thanks to these special policies, the impoverished areas have seen significant improvement in the production and living conditions and the development of human capital, while the poverty-stricken people have been empowered to shake off poverty and get rich by their own efforts.

1.2.3 Remarkable Improvement in Production and Living Conditions in Poverty-Stricken Areas

Since the launch of MDGs in 2000, China has carried out the *Development-Oriented Poverty Reduction for China's Rural Areas (2001–2010) and the Outline for Development-Oriented Poverty Reduction for China's Rural Areas (2011–2020)*, leading to remarkable improvement in the infrastructure, public services and people's life in the poverty-stricken areas.

The impoverished areas have seen continuous improvement in infrastructure. By the end of 2015, 99.7% of natural villages in these areas gained access to power supply, 97.6% had telephone access, 56.3% had broadband access, 73.0% had tarmac or cement trunk roads and 47.8% had access to bus services.[13]

The people's life has improved markedly as well. A rising proportion of the rural residents in poverty-stricken areas have gained access to main durable goods. By 2015, every 100 rural households owned 8.3 cars, 75.6 washing machines, 67.6 refrigerators, 208.9 mobile phones, and 13.2 computers. In addition, 99.8% of rural households had access to electric lighting, 61.5% to piped water, 85.3% had no difficulty with access to drinking water and 93.6% had their own toilets.[14]

1.2.4 Rising Education Level of the Poor People

The 2014 statistics on basic education in China showed that the enrollment rate stood at 97.3% for children aged 7–12 in poverty-stricken rural areas, 97.6% for those aged 13–15, and 72.5% for those aged 3–5 in kindergartens. The dropout rate for the under 16 was 0.3%, among which 21.8% dropped out of primary schools, 63.5% out of junior high school and 14.7% out of senior high school. The girls' right to compulsory education had been effectively guaranteed. In 2014, the enrollment rate reached 97.4% for girls aged 7–12 in poverty-stricken rural areas, 97.7% for

[13]Department of Household Surveys of National Bureau of Statistics (2016).

[14]Department of Household Surveys of National Bureau of Statistics (2016).

those aged 13–15, compared with 97.1 and 97.5%, respectively, for boys of the same age group.[15]

Vocational education has developed to be an important way to improve the human capital of poor families and prevent the intergenerational transmission of poverty. To help with the employment of young people from poverty-stricken families, the State Council Leading Group Office of Poverty Alleviation and Development and the Ministry of Finance have actively promoted the Dewdrop Project since 2004. With the focus on improving the capacity for self-development and boosting employment of the poor population, the project is mainly supported by government funds for poverty reduction and encourages the participation of all sectors of society. It boosts the employment and work-based earnings of the poor population through a package of special measures for poverty reduction, such as financing and guiding the poor rural labors to receive vocational education and various skills training, nurturing the leaders for industrial development in poverty-stricken villages, among others.

1.2.5 Constantly Improving Social Safety Net in Poverty-Stricken Areas

The Chinese government attaches great importance to the construction of social safety net in poverty-stricken areas. The social security system has been established and improved, incorporating subsistence allowances, relief and support system for people living in dire poverty, relief for victims of natural disasters, assistance in medical care, education, housing and employment, temporary relief, just to name a few. The system of "Five Guarantees" (for food, clothing, medical care, housing and burial expenses) has been improved to guarantee the basic life needs of the rural residents with no working ability. By the end of 2015, the urban subsistence allowances benefited 9,574,000 households of 17,011,000 people, and the rural subsistence allowances were delivered to 28,462,000 households of 49,036,000 people.[16] The system of subsistence allowances plays an important role in the social safety net.

The impoverished areas have witnessed sustained improvement in the conditions for medical care. The healthcare service system of the state-level hospitals in rural China has continued to improve. The proportion of administrative villages with clinics went up from 89.8% in 2000 to 94.1% in 2014, and the proportion of the people in impoverished rural areas with access to timely medical treatment reached 94.4% in 2014.[17] The New Rural Cooperative Medical System has achieved full coverage and the community-level healthcare service system has been continuously improved. In today's rural China, the problem of "unaffordable and unavailable medical care" has been greatly eased and the life expectancy of the poor has risen steadily.

---

[15]Department of Household Surveys of National Bureau of Statistics (2016).

[16]Source: statistics from the official website of the Ministry of Civil Affairs. http://www.mca.gov.cn/.

[17]Department of Household Surveys of National Bureau of Statistics (2016).

1.3 China's Contribution to Global Poverty Reduction

China's experience has contributed to global poverty reduction in both theory and practice.

1.3.1 Theoretical Contribution

The twenty-first century has come with profound changes in global economy and international relations. Following the financial crisis in 2008 in particular, the dominant position of developed countries has changed and the emerging economies, especially the BRICS countries, have risen to become the mainstay of global economic growth. China's practical experience in poverty reduction provides a wealth of materials for researchers in various fields. Researchers and research institutes in economics, sociology, international relations, diplomacy, development and other disciplines have updated their system of knowledge based on China's practices.

1. A new understanding of the government–market relationship

China's primary experience in poverty reduction is to "stick to government leadership and enhance government responsibility." This poses challenges to traditional development theory, one of which lies in the government–market relationship in poverty-reduction project. The traditional development theory based on market economy holds that the main culprit for economic backwardness in the impoverished areas is the lack of an effective market mechanism. That also explains why the World Bank and IMF have been promoting the Washington Consensus to developing countries. However, the facts demonstrate that the complete reliance on the market only widens the gap between rich and poor and undermines the foundation of poverty reduction.

The "government leadership" in China's poverty-reduction projects differs from the government's planning and intervention in the market as stressed by the "old" structural economics. In the process of developing "special economic zones" and labor-intensive manufacturing industries, China took full advantage of globalization and market mechanism to ideally allocate and utilize its resource endowments. It advocates a development model that pays more respect to the market–government combination. It does not rely too much on government intervention as advocated by traditional structural economics, nor does it leave all to the market as promoted by the Washington Consensus. The government intervention should be best illustrated through the "identification" and "facilitation" in the process of industrial upgrading and technological innovation.[18]

Chinese government has played a central role in poverty reduction all along. It sees it as the innate call of the socialist system to eradicate poverty, improve people's wellbeing and achieve common prosperity. The government plays a leading role in

---

[18] Lin (2012a, b, 2014).

eradicating poverty. Instead of laying overall responsibility on the government, such government-led model of poverty reduction draws on the joint efforts of government, society and the market through clear strategies, plans and policy system on poverty reduction. The government is mainly responsible for formulating strategies and continuously innovating and improving the policy system, so as to make the policies governing economic and social development more inclusive and more beneficial to the poor. The government makes continued efforts to foster infrastructure development in poverty-stricken areas and improve public services. By giving priority to issues relating to agriculture, rural areas and rural people, the government has laid an increasingly solid foundation for poverty reduction. By creating a business environment favorable for the transfer of employment in poverty-stricken areas, the government has opened up more channels to increase the income of the poor. Moreover, the government has kept improving the social security policies to ensure the basic and subsistence needs of those most in need. Such government-led model of poverty reduction has been recognized by international scholars.

2. Actively promote international development cooperation in poverty reduction

It can be seen from the previous section on the developed countries' role and actions in MDGs that the traditional donors, despite their active part in relevant MDGs initiatives, have been slow in fulfilling their commitments with sluggish aids. MDGs have evolved into a game of "money from rich countries and actions from poor countries."[19]

Poverty reduction in China distinguishes itself from that in other developing countries which received large amounts of international development assistance. In China's development financing, the international development assistance only makes up a small proportion. The key contributor to development should be China's market financing mechanism that makes the best use of FDI and international trade. In the early days of reform and opening up, China was short of development capital. As a recipient country, China worked hard to secure international development assistance, while improving management methods, agricultural technology, and monitoring and evaluation in the process of utilizing foreign investment. For instance, the biggest gain from the World Bank's poverty reduction project in China has been more about the project management experience than the agricultural products it produces, which helped China develop and improve its own project management methods.

Xiaolin Wang and Qianqian Liu studied the theoretical basis of China's poverty-reduction model and made the following conclusions. Assistance, as a public product, should give full play to the leading role of the government. In terms of investment and trade, the private sector should be encouraged to play a role to attract investment to the recipient country and improve local productivity, while boosting international trade and connecting the recipient country's domestic market with the global economy. Such model is conducive to enhancing the country's capabilities that constitute the foundation for socioeconomic development and poverty reduction.[20]

[19]Simon (2014).

[20]Wang and Liu (2012).

Guided by such development philosophy, China–Africa cooperation successfully facilitated the development and poverty reduction in Africa. Traditional international aid for development is granted on the condition of national democratization, thus excluding the countries most in need which are typically poor in democratization, and leading to the loss and waste of assistance.[21] Africa is a developing region and China is a developing country. At the macro level, China provides assistance to Africa for infrastructure development in transportation, agriculture, water conservancy and others, creating external conditions for the regional economic growth. At the micro level, China encourages the companies to go global, make investment and conduct trade in Africa in a bid to energize the market and create a large number of accessible jobs for the young people so that they can thrive on their own. Such growth-oriented China–Africa cooperation, different from the process-oriented OECD-DAC assistance, sets up a more open and inclusive model for South–South cooperation.[22]

3. Take an active part in global poverty governance

Since its accession to the WTO in 2001, China has been a strong advocate of global free trade, attaching importance to developing win–win partnerships. China has repeatedly called for building an "interconnected" international community with shared future for mankind, advocating a new thinking of win–win and all-win cooperation, and discarding the old mentality of zero-sum game or winner taking all, which epitomized China's wisdom and values conducive to global governance. In fact, such philosophy has been based on the successful practice of eradicating poverty through cooperation in the process of globalization since the launch of reform and opening-up in China. In this way, China is helping improve the global poverty governance.

At the beginning of the MDGs, the developed and developing countries—the subjects for the attainment of MDGs—were viewed as two independent and opposite camps, which is inconsistent with the status-quo of international relations. The process toward the adoption of Sustainable Development Goals (SDGs) suggested that the advancing globalization posed new challenges to the traditional bipolar system of the world. The dependence between developed and developing countries is no longer one-way: their relationship has become a highly interdependent "cobweb relationship," featuring co-dependence and mutual influence among each other. In this connection, the cooperation between developed and developing countries should no longer be based on a donor–recipient relationship, but toward a win–win result. The main body of global development should be more diversified and inclusive, opening up channels to get enterprises, non-governmental organizations and the public more involved. We should give full play to the initiative of each player and strengthen cooperation to build a new type of partnership. "Time for Global Action" has been a rallying call since the launch of SDGs, for which China has been an excellent case in point with its own development, particularly the Belt and Road Initiative it proposed.

---

[21] Li (2014).

[22] Department of Household Surveys of National Bureau of Statistics (2016).

1.3.2 Practical Contribution

1. Significant drop of the global poor population

China's achievements in poverty reduction have made tremendous contribution to the global poverty reduction by pushing for the attainment of MDGs and the steady improvement of Human Development Index (HDI). Measured against the World Bank's poverty line of USD 1.25 a day (2005 PPP), the global poor population dropped by 1,090 million, from 1,926 million in 1990 to 836 million in 2015. Over the same period, the poor population in China decreased by 635 million, from 690 million to 55 million, accounting for 58.25% of the global poverty reduction. Between 1981 and 2015 China contributed 70% of global poverty reduction.

As to its contribution to the global HDI improvement—HDI is a composite index of income, education, life expectancy, among others, used to measure the socioeconomic development of countries—China's HDI increased swiftly by 44.8% from 0.502 in 1990 to 0.727 in 2015, as against 19.1% from 0.597 to 0.711 globally. China's poverty-reduction progress has been highly acclaimed by the international community. In an article published in the *People's Daily* Overseas Edition on October 24, 2011, the author Helen Clark, then-administrator of UNDP, wrote that "China is exerting a more crucial impact on sustainable global economic growth and the development of the Millennium Development Goals through its decisions and actions than ever before. The United Nations must work with the Chinese government to achieve the goals of reducing poverty in China and the rest of the world as well as promoting green, inclusive and sustainable development across the globe."[23]

2. A model for reference to other developing countries

China's poverty-reduction model, though not replicable, delivers valuable lessons for economic transition and poverty elimination in other developing countries. In December 2007 Lennart Båge, then-President of the International Fund for Agricultural Development (IFAD), said in an interview with Xinhua News Agency at the IFAD headquarters in Rome that thanks to the reform and opening up over the past 30 years, China made astonishing achievements in agricultural development and poverty reduction that other developing countries can draw experience from. According to the "Economic Transformation and Poverty Reduction: How It Happened in China, Helping It Happen in Africa (Policy Report)" published by China-DAC Study Group in 2012, the Chinese experience has once again shown that against the backdrop of globalization, the emergence of a growth-oriented powerful leadership with a focus on development rather than deep-rooted policies and interests will bring about rapid socioeconomic development in poor countries. In this

[23]Clark (2011).

context, the national economic transformation could succeed within a single generation, which would motivate and mobilize united efforts of the whole nation. Africa has much to learn from Chinese experience.[24]

3. A catalyst for policy reforms in other developing countries

China's achievements in poverty reduction have inspired a rash of new experiments in some active countries, such as the experiment with special economic zones (SEZs) which could be divided into three categories: free economic zones (FTZs), export processing zones (EPZs) and multi-purpose zones (MPZ). SEZs could reduce poverty directly by creating jobs and indirectly by attracting FDI in relevant industries.

Most African countries set up SEZs between the late 1990s and the first decade of the twenty-first century. The SEZs in many countries, such as Ethiopia, Kenya and Ghana, mainly feature the local industries facing global economic competition, like clothing, textile and agricultural products.[25] At the first Ministerial Conference of the Forum on China–Africa Cooperation in 2000, China pledged to share its experience in boosting investment and improving management through SEZs. During the third edition of the Ministerial Conference in 2006, then-President Jintao Hu announced to set up three to five SEZs in Africa. Subsequently, such SEZs were successively established in Zambia, Egypt, Nigeria, Ethiopia and Mauritius. Studies by International Poverty Reduction Center in China and UNDP show that China's experience in SEZs development could be a guide for African countries to establish SEZs in line with their national conditions. It's advisable to avoid single-industry SEZs and encourage various sectors to invest in the SEZs in a bid to form an industrial chain conducive to the national economic growth.[26] African governments should try their best to integrate resources to put in place safe and convenient infrastructure as well as preferential policies in customs, taxation and recruitment for investing enterprises, in a bid to leverage open and inclusive policies to attract enterprises to invest in Africa.

1.4 Conclusions and Discussion

The MDGs effectively forged a global consensus and garnered attention and recognition from all over the world. It is one of the most important political commitment documents for international development in today's world. It unleashed humanity's courage to meet the challenge of eradicating poverty, and delivered spectacular results.

The Chinese government has responded positively to the Millennium Declaration. By formulating poverty-reduction strategies suited to the national conditions and implementing feasible plans, China became the first country to achieve the goal of

[24]China-DAC Study Group (2012).

[25]Farole (2011).

[26]International Poverty Reduction Center in China, and UNDP (2015).

halving the poor population and made outstanding contributions to the attainment of MDGs. China's achievements in poverty reduction are multifaceted. Between 1990 and 2015, the proportion of people whose income is less than USD 1.25 a day fell from 74 to 4%, that of malnourished people also dropped significantly, the education and health development index improved substantially, and the living standards measured against access to electricity, drinking water, durable goods and others rose markedly.

China's contribution to global poverty reduction mainly comes down to the following points.

First, China explored a development-oriented poverty-reduction path befitting its national circumstances. While adhering to the government leadership and strengthening the government responsibility, China highly values the role of market mechanism. In the process of globalization, China gave full play to the resources' endowments and comparative advantages. The public policies to benefit the poverty-stricken areas and population have been introduced to facilitate pro-poor growth and inclusive development. A solid foundation for poverty reduction has been laid by safeguarding agriculture, rural areas and farmers as the core. Constant efforts have been made to create a market environment conducive to the employment transfer of labor forces in poverty-stricken areas, increasing their income sources. Furthermore, the social security system has seen continuous improvement to ensure the basic and subsistence needs of those most in need.

Second, China explored new concepts and approaches for international cooperation in poverty reduction. As China's practice of poverty reduction posed challenges to traditional development concepts, a growing number of scholars at home and abroad began to analyze China's practices from different perspectives, triggering economists' rethinking about the roles of government and market, the new insights of international relations scholars into South–South Cooperation and a new type of China–Africa partnership, just to name a few. As the discussions over an increasing number of views continue to rage, we can rest assured that there is more than one answer and more than one path for development. What matters most is to find a development path best suited to the national conditions.

Third, China provides a model for reference to other developing countries. China's poverty-reduction model, though not replicable, delivers valuable lessons for economic transition and poverty elimination in other developing countries. China's experience is multifaceted. Based on China's model, other developing countries could develop their own models and approaches in line with domestic needs and priorities of development. China's experience in poverty reduction is a vast treasure trove for the rest of the world.

References

China-DAC Study Group.(2012). Economic transformation and poverty reduction how It happened in China, helping It happen in Africa (Policy Report). China Financial and Economic Publishing House.

Clark, H. (2011). Sharing China's poverty reduction experience. In *People's daily* (Overseas ed).

Department of Household Surveys of National Bureau of Statistics. (2016). Poverty Monitoring Report of Rural China 2015 (pp. 13–21), China Statistics Press.

Farole, T. (2011). *Special economic zones in Africa: comparing performance and learning from global experience. Directions in development*. Washington, D.C: World Bank.

Huang, C. W. (2016). New development Philosophies and poverty reduction project. *The Forum of Leadership Science, 4.*

IFPRI. (2015). 2015 Global hunger index armed conflict and the challenge of hunger. International Food Policy Research Institute.

International Poverty Reduction Center in China, and UNDP. (2015). If Africa builds nests, will the birds come?—Comparative study on special economic zones in Africa and China. International Poverty Reduction Center in China Research Reports, 6.

Li, D. (2014). new ideas and new model: China's contributions to the reform of international development. *Journal of Xiamen University (Arts and Social Sciences), 4.*

Lin, J. Y. (2012a). *The quest for prosperity: How developing economies can take off* (pp. 171–183, Z. Jianhua, Trans.). Beijing: Beijing University Press.

Lin, J. Y. (2012b). *New structural economics* (pp. 15–17, S. Jian, Trans.). Beijing: Beijing University Press.

Lin, J. Y. (2014). *New structural economics: A framework for rethinking development and policy* (pp. 1–20, S. Jian, Trans.). Beijing: Beijing University Press.

Ministry of Foreign Affairs of People's Republic of China and United Nations in China. (2015). Report on China's implementation of the millennium development goals (2000–2015).

OECD. (2005). The paris declaration on aid effectiveness: Five principles for smart aid. http://www.oecd.org/dac/effectiveness/45827300.pdf.

Simon, B. (2014). Development goals: Tackling poverty's root causes. Swissinfo. https://www.swissinfo.ch/chi/politics/下一步_发展目标-解决贫困的根源问题/40600040.

UN. (2002). Implementation of the United Nations Millennium Declaration (Report of the Secretary-General), Fifty-seventh session, Item 44 of the provisional agenda.

UN. (2005). *Investing in development: A practical plan to achieve the millennium development goals.*

UN. (2015). The millennium development goals report 2015, UN research report.

UN Millennium Project. (2005). *Investing in development: A practical plan to achieve the millennium development goals*. New York.

United Nations. (2001). Road map towards the implementation of the United Nations Millennium Declaration, A/56/326.

Wang, X., & Liu Q. (2012). China-Africa cooperation: A new way to improve development effectiveness. *International Studies, 5.*

Chapter 2
SDGs in Poverty Reduction: Substance and Policy Options

The first goal of the Sustainable Development Goals (SDGs) is to "end poverty in all its forms everywhere," making it clear that eradication of extreme poverty serves as the foundation for sustainable development, and extreme poverty should be eradicated through sustainable development. The main target of MDGs in poverty reduction is to halve the proportion of people whose income is less than one dollar a day. In compassion, the goal of "ending poverty in all its forms" in SDGs expanded the dimensions of poverty and elevated the international community's understanding of poverty to a higher level. The policies lay more stress on equal rights to economic resources, access to basic services, ownership and control of properties, among others. These new ideas went beyond the traditional definition of poverty as "basic needs" for survival, featuring the new contents about understanding and ending poverty through "basic capabilities" for development. This chapter begins with an analysis of the contents, relations and policy orientation of the targets under SDGs in poverty reduction, followed by a study of the system framework that needs to be put in place or improved for the attainment of the targets, before putting forward proposals to improve China's poverty-reduction strategies and policies in light of the UN poverty-reduction goals by 2030. The Chinese government is advised to, between 2021 and 2030, set multidimensional poverty standards on the basis of "basic needs" and "basic capabilities" approaches, so as to fully identify and assess "poverty in all forms." It's advised to further improve the economic security, public services and social security system for the poor people, empower them to be more resilient against economic, social, environmental shocks and disasters, and eradicate poverty through sustainable development.

X. Wang and X. Zhang, *Towards 2030 – China's Poverty Alleviation and Global Poverty Governance*, International Research on Poverty Reduction,
https://doi.org/10.1007/978-981-15-6356-0_2

2.1 Poverty-Reduction Targets: Substance and Connections

The 2030 Agenda for Sustainable Development[1] was initiated by the UN and adopted by world leaders on 25 September 2015 at the United Nations Sustainable Development Summit. Among the 17 SDGs of the 2030 Agenda for Sustainable Development, the first goal is to "end poverty in all forms everywhere." The priority in the ensuing 15 years is to fulfil the goal of ending poverty in all forms and achieving sustainable

Table 2.1 Targets of SDGs in Poverty Reduction

GOAL 1: End poverty in all its forms everywhere	
Targets	
1.1	By 2030, eradicate extreme poverty for all people everywhere, currently measured as people living on less than USD 1.25 a day
1.2	By 2030, reduce at least by half the proportion of men, women and children of all ages living in poverty in all its forms according to national definitions
1.3	Implement nationally appropriate social protection systems and measures for all, including floors, and by 2030 achieve substantial coverage of the poor and the vulnerable
1.4	By 2030, ensure that all men and women, in particular the poor and the vulnerable, have equal rights to economic resources, as well as access to basic services, ownership and control over land and other forms of property, inheritance, natural resources, appropriate new technology and financial services, including microfinance
1.5	By 2030, build the resilience of the poor and those in vulnerable situations and reduce their exposure and vulnerability to climate-related extreme events and other economic, social and environmental shocks and disasters
1.A	Ensure significant mobilization of resources from a variety of sources, including through enhanced development cooperation, in order to provide adequate and predictable means for developing countries, in particular least developed countries, to implement programmes and policies to end poverty in all its forms
1.B	Create sound policy frameworks at the national, regional and international levels, based on pro-poor and gender-sensitive development strategies, to support accelerated investment in poverty eradication actions

Source The UN Sustainable Development Goals

[1]The 2030 Agenda for Sustainable Development is built on a series of preliminary outcomes. Among them, the most important reports include Realizing the Future We Want for All and A Renewed Global Partnership for Development released successively in June 2012 and March 2013 by the UN System Task Team on the Post-2015 UN Development Agenda (UNSTT), A New Global Partnership: Eradicate Poverty and Transform Economies through Sustainable Development submitted in May 2013 by High Level Panel of Eminent Persons on the Post-2015 Development Agenda (HLP), Report of the Open Working Group on Sustainable Development Goals issued in September 2014 by the UNGA Open Working Group on Sustainable Development Goals (the Open Working Group in short), and The Road to Dignity by 2030: Ending Poverty, Transforming All Lives and Protecting the Planet—Synthesis Report of the Secretary-General on the Post-2015 Agenda to all member states at the end of 2014.

development by 2030 through united efforts of governments, international organizations, civil societies and others. The goal is subdivided into five targets as shown in Table 2.1.

The above five targets fall into three categories. The first category, comprising 1.1 and 1.2, sets the targets for poverty reduction. The second category, covering 1.3, 1.4 and 1.5, establishes the domestic institutional framework for the attainment of poverty-reduction targets. The third category, including 1.A and 1.B, puts forward a policy framework of international development cooperation for the attainment of poverty-reduction targets.

2.1.1 Poverty-Reduction Targets

The first two targets in poverty reduction, to be achieved by 2030, are set by the UN. Target 1.1 is to eradicate extreme poverty for all people everywhere by 2030, measured as people living on less than USD 1.25 a day (2005 PPP). In October 2015, the World Bank updated the global line to USD 1.9 a day (2011 PPP). That is to say, as of 2030, the extreme poverty measured as people living on less than USD 1.9 a day will be eradicated everywhere. This is a mandatory target for global poverty reduction. Target 1.2 is to reduce, by 2030, at least by half the proportion of men, women and children of all ages living in poverty in all its forms according to national definitions.

2.1.2 Domestic System

Targets 1.3, 1.4 and 1.5 are essentially the domestic poverty-reduction system required for the attainment of targets 1.1 and 1.2. First, implement social protection system with substantial coverage of the poor and the vulnerable. Second, ensure all people have equal rights to economic resources, as well as access to basic services, ownership and control over land and other forms of property, inheritance, natural resources appropriate new technology and financial services, including microfinance. Third, build the resilience of the poor and those in vulnerable situations and reduce their exposure and vulnerability to climate-related extreme events and other economic, social and environmental shocks and disasters.

2.1.3 Fundraising and International Cooperation

"A variety of sources" in target 1.A include government, market, social organizations, private sector and others at home, as well as international development cooperation. As developing countries, especially low-income countries, have difficulty in achieving the UN's poverty-reduction goals on their own, the UN proposed the international development cooperation policies as stated in targets 1.A and 1.B, emphasizing to increase investment in international development through international development cooperation to provide schemes, policies and funds for the eradication of extreme poverty in developing countries.

2.2 Understanding and Assessing Poverty in All Its Forms

2.2.1 Meaning of "Poverty in All Its Forms"

To "end poverty in all its forms" is a giant leap in human understanding of poverty. The countries and international organizations used to define poverty as measured against such indicators as income or consumption. The poverty line was defined as the amount of money needed to purchase "a basket" of goods and services at market price to meet the basic needs for living. The people without enough money for such basic needs are defined as the poor population. The poverty line defined on the basis of income (or consumption) provides useful information, but far from the poor people's feelings and situations in reality. With 109 francs and 15 sous in his pocket, Jean Valjean, the protagonist in the renowned novel *Les Misérables*, still suffered from hunger and cold. Due to his "identity," he's socially excluded and couldn't find himself a shelter. There's more to poverty than income. We have enough reason to believe that the "poverty in all its forms" refers to both the lack of income to meet the basic needs and the hardships from the lack of access to basic education, medical service, housing, employment and others. We need to understand poverty in all its forms from the following dimensions. First, poor people can experience many different forms of deprivation at the same time and each form is important.[2] Second, no single-dimension measure of poverty could match with the multidimensional poverty. For instance, the studies on India and Peru suggested that many people with poor capabilities in education, health and other aspects are not poor in terms of income. Third, income is a good proxy variable for multidimensional poverty, but not capable of reflecting the deprivation and social exclusion in other aspects. Fourth, the multidimensional measures of poverty could direct public policy to the fields that need primary intervention. Fifth, the multidimensional measure of poverty is an important supplement, rather than substitute, to the indicator of income. *Pin–kun*, The Chinese equivalent of "poverty," is more profound and accurate. The income indicator could help measure the "lack of income," and the indicators in other dimensions could point to the "hardships."[3]

---

[2]Sen (1992).

[3]Wang (2017).

2.2.2 Measurement of Poverty in All Its Forms

Following the proposed goal of "ending poverty in all its forms everywhere" for the 2030 Agenda for Sustainable Development, the debate about the measurement of poverty in all its forms raged fiercely. Under the leadership of Sabina Alkire, the Multidimensional Poverty Peer Network (MPPN, the official website: http://www.mppn.org) convened experts and scholars for lobbying at the UN's side events on sustainable development and statistics. MPPN believes that it's difficult to capture real poverty in line with the poverty line of USD 1.25 a day (consumption-based poverty). The Multidimensional Poverty Index (MPI) is the most appropriate measure of multidimensional poverty. It could be applied to measure most of the SDGs indicators on hunger, nutrition, health, education and others relating to human development.

However, in the statement of the five targets under the SDGs in poverty reduction, it wasn't explicitly stated to apply MPI to measure poverty in all its forms. Target 1.1—2030, eradicate extreme poverty for all people everywhere, currently measured as people living on less than USD 1.25 a day"—sets the standard for global extreme poverty. Target 1.2—"by 2030, reduce at least by half the proportion of men, women and children of all ages living in poverty in all its forms according to national definitions"—states how to evaluate poverty in all its forms. The specific policies to define and measure "poverty in all its forms" are left to the state government to formulate on their own, which is a linchpin to end poverty in all its forms everywhere by 2030. In this sense, it is of paramount importance to raise awareness of poverty measurement and promote the application of MPI to poverty reduction in all countries.

2.2.3 Combination of Basic Needs with Basic Capabilities to Measure Poverty in All Its Forms

The existing definitions and measurements of poverty fall into two categories. One category is based on the theory about basic needs, defining poverty as a deprivation of basic needs caused by a lack of income or wealth. In this way, the definition of extreme poverty depends on that of basic needs, including food and non-food needs. The amount of money required to meet such basic needs is defined as a line for income-based or consumption-based poverty.[4] The World Bank set the extreme poverty line at USD 1.25 a day per person (2005 PPP) based on the theory about basic needs for human survival and the median poverty line of 15 low-income countries.

The other category is based on the theory about basic capabilities. Amartya Sen pointed out that we have good reason to believe that poverty is the deprivation of basic capabilities rather than lowness of incomes. Deprivation of basic capabilities could be manifested as premature death, significant malnutrition (especially for children),

[4]For detailed discussions in this respect, see *The Measurement of Poverty: Theories and Methods* by Xiaoling Wang published by Social Sciences Academic Press in 2017.

persistent morbidity, widespread illiteracy and other deficiencies.[5] Alkire and Foster put forward with AF method for MPI measurement based on the theory about basic capabilities and use it to evaluate multidimensional poverty. The UNDP adopted the global multidimensional poverty index measured with AF method and began to publish the global multidimensional poverty situation in the annual Human Development Report since 2010. The global MPI assesses poverty from three dimensions: education, health and living standards, incorporating 10 indicators. It complements the World Bank's income-based (or consumption-based) poverty line. To achieve the goal of "by 2030, reducing at least by half the proportion of men, women and children of all ages living in poverty in all its forms according to national definitions," I believe that each country needs to develop their own multidimensional poverty indicators to measure "poverty in all its forms."

To eradicate poverty in all its manifestations, it's necessary to integrate the existing poverty measurement theories by combining the income-based poverty line based on the theory about basic needs with the MPI based on the theory about basic capabilities, so as to measure both the "insufficiency" of income and the "hardships" in other aspects. Only by doing so we can have a powerful tool for poverty measurement. Economists generally assume that the shopping basket for the measurement of income-based poverty covers food and non-food basic needs, both measurable in amount of money. However, the fact is that in numerous poverty-stricken mountain villages, the absence of primary school made education for children there quite difficult, while the absence of clinics made it difficult for people to seek medical treatment. Such basic public services that should be provided by the government cannot be purchased by individuals. China's poverty-reduction goal of "two no-worries and three guarantees" is based on a multidimensional view of poverty. When the goal is achieved, those who have been living in poverty no longer have to worry about food and clothing, and they would have guaranteed access to compulsory education, basic medical treatment and housing. In May 2016, the General Office of the Communist Party of China Central Committee and the General Office of the State Council issued the *Opinions on Establishing a Poverty Delisting Mechanism.* The household-based mechanism makes it clear that the registered families would be removed from the poor register if they have a stable annual per capita net income above the national poverty line, and guaranteed access to food, clothing, compulsory education, basic medical service and housing. This criterion is based on the concept of multidimensional poverty and China's reality, taking into account both income and such measures as food, clothing and access to compulsory education, basic medical services, and housing. It could be used to evaluate the progress toward the goal of ending poverty in all its forms by 2020.

[5] Sen (2000).

2.3 Pro-poor Universal Social Protection Systems

The poverty-reduction target 1.3 proposes to "implement nationally appropriate social protection systems and measures for all, including floors, and by 2030 achieve substantial coverage of the poor and the vulnerable." According to the United Nations Research Institute for Social Development (UNRISD), social protection is concerned with preventing, managing and overcoming situations that adversely affect people's wellbeing.[6] According to the World Bank, social protection consists of policies and programs designed to reduce poverty and vulnerability by promoting efficient labor markets, diminishing people's exposure to risks, and enhancing their capacity to manage economic and social risks, such as unemployment, exclusion, sickness, disability and old age.[7] The social protection mainly takes the form of labor market intervention, social insurance and social assistance.

The above target 1.3 was set up to urge countries to establish systems for labor market intervention, social insurance and social assistance, mainly targeting the poor and the vulnerable. In China, for example, the social protection systems should at least incorporate the following contents: the social assistance system for the poor, such as the subsistence allowance system; the social protection system for the vulnerable group of children, such as orphans, de facto unattended children, street children and left-behind children; the system to provide subsidies, assistance and caring for rural and urban elders, in particular the disabled ones; the social protection system for vulnerable groups, such as ethnic minorities and women; as well as the universal medical insurance system and medical assistance system.

It's undoubtedly the common aspiration of all low-income countries and all people in extreme poverty to establish a subsistence allowance system with full coverage of the poor and the vulnerable. In fact, however, many developing countries established the poverty-reduction system based on income support modeled on the social welfare system of the Western developed countries. It has turned out that these countries didn't progress well in poverty reduction as expected, due to the insufficient national financial resources. China has been following the path of combining development-oriented with social-security-based poverty reduction. The development-oriented poverty reduction focuses on the development of production capacity and conditions in impoverished areas as well as the production and living capacities of the poor people. Should China's poverty-reduction policies only focus on social protection or income support, there would be a great financial burden on the country, in addition to the phenomenon of "supporting the lazy ones." Should China's poverty-reduction policies focus on development alone, the poor population would not be able to enjoy social protection policies for the access to education, medical treatment and pensions, which would make it quite difficult to get rid of poverty.

There was a poverty-stricken family surnamed Yao in JH village, RJ county of Guizhou Province in southwest China. This family of ethnic Miao has four members, Yao who is 30 years old, his 67-year-old mother who has lost the ability to work

[6] United Nations Research Institute for Social Development (UNRISD) (2010).

[7] World Bank (2001).

and two daughters of 6 and 8 years old. Prior to 2014, the family lived a difficult but not impoverished life. Yao, his wife and his mother managed to feed the family with about 1,900 m^2 of farmland and 3,000 m^2 of forest land. In 2014, Yao and his wife left the hometown for work. Speaking poor *putonghua* and with insufficient education, they could only find some rough work to do, but still they could bring more than RMB 3,000 home for a half year. In 2015, Yao's mother fell ill and lost the ability to work. Yao's wife had to stay at home to take care of Yao's mother. Moreover, since there is only kindergarten in the village, but not primary school, Yao's wife had to shuttle her first daughter back and forth between the school in the township and home, and her younger daughter between kindergarten in the village and home. Feeling hopeless and desperate, Yao's wife abandoned the family (without going through the divorce), leaving the responsibility to Yao alone to support the family of four. Without enough farmland and unable to go out for work, Yao's family fell into extreme poverty.

In 2015, Yao's family was registered as a poverty-stricken household. An officer from the township government took up the responsibility for helping the family. At the time, the pork could be sold for a good price and Yao hoped to raise 10 pigs but had no fund or technology. The officer helped him get a small loan from poverty-reduction programs and provided him with technical training. In this way, Yao could raise pigs at home while taking care of his mother and daughters, in addition to a certain amount of cash income. The family is expected to shake off poverty by 2017.

Source: An interview done by the author on May 6, 2015.

China has since 2002 begun to establish the New Rural Cooperative Medical System (NRCMS), featuring the comprehensive management of serious disease insurance. The rural subsistence allowance system set up in 2006, the social old-age insurance system in 2009, nine-year compulsory education system and other social protection and public service systems have proved crucial for the elimination of extreme poverty. Family Yao's situation could have gone worse without the help of these systems. Thanks to the nine-year compulsory education system, Yao's daughters could go to school, preventing the intergenerational transmission of poverty. Thanks to the rural social old-age insurance system, Yao's mother got cash income. Without the safety net weaved by the social protection systems, the intergenerational transmission of poverty would be highly likely. Currently, China needs to systematically assess and test the pro-poor nature of the social protection systems, so that such systems could play a significant role in eliminating poverty, narrowing development gap and enhancing social cohesion.

2.4 Equal Rights to Economic Resources and Basic Services

Poverty-reduction target 1.4 proposed to "by 2030, ensure that all men and women, in particular the poor and the vulnerable, have equal rights to economic resources, as well as access to basic services, ownership and control over land and other forms of property, inheritance, natural resources, appropriate new technology and financial

Table 2.2 Economic entitlement system relating to poverty reduction

Type of rights	Policy instrument
Production-based entitlements	• Use of land and natural resources • Subsidies to producers • Tax breaks • Support for production credit
Trade-based entitlements	• Free-exchange market • "Fair trade" for the poor
Own-labor entitlements	• Fair employment • Provide job as a form of relief • Free flow of population
Inheritance and transfer entitlements	• Inheritance and transfer of property and legacy

services, including microfinance." To achieve the 2030 Sustainable Development Goals as scheduled, it's important to understand the role of economic rights and public services in poverty reduction.

Amartya Sen stressed that "starvation is the characteristic of some people not having enough food to eat. It is not the characteristic of there being not enough food to eat. Food supply statements say things about a commodity (or a group of commodities) considered on its own. Starvation statements are about the relationship of persons to the commodity (or that commodity group). Starvation statements translate readily into statements of ownership of food by persons. Ownership relations are one kind of entitlement relations. It's necessary to understand the entitlement systems within which the problem of starvation is to be analyzed."[8] Based on Amartya Sen's theory about poverty and entitlements and in combination with the target 1.4, the author made the following economic entitlement system relating to poverty reduction (see Table 2.2).

Between 1981 and 2015, China lifted over 700 million people living on less than USD 1.9 a day out of poverty. A fundamental lesson from the experience is to give full play to the key role of inclusive and pro-poor rural land system. Through the reform of rural land contracting system, the farmers got the production-based and the own-labor entitlements. China's basic national conditions feature a large population with relatively little (arable) land, with the per capita arable land of less than 0.1 hectare. To eliminate poverty or to provide enough food for the Chinese people under such circumstances, we should first solve the entitlement relation between people and land, before addressing the technical problems. It's also why generations of Chinese policymakers have all regarded the land system reform as a key to national stability. As for economic entitlement, the most important one for poverty elimination is the poor people's right to acquire and use the land. In China's policy system for targeted poverty reduction, there's still great space for improvement concerning the poor people's access to valued-added income from land and natural resources.

[8] Amartya Sen (2001).

Improvement in this regard would be crucial and plays a well-leveraged role to ensure the sustained and steady effect of poverty reduction.

Another issue that matters is the inclusive financial service. Land, labor and capital are the most important factors of production. Most developing countries, in particular the low-income countries, have a surplus of labors. Assuming that the poor people have the entitlements to use the land, another key factor for poverty elimination would be the access to capital. The productivity could be increased with an effective combination of land, labor and capital. In fact, however, the poverty-stricken areas and people are often in the vicious cycle of "poverty traps," with difficult access to capital. The poor people could gain capital from two sources: the poverty-reduction fund, including domestic government budget for poverty reduction and the ODA from other countries; and financial funds, including small loans and mutual aid funds for poverty reduction. The first one is public fund and the lower the income level, the less money the government has and the less allocated for poverty reduction. Therefore, the key to eliminating poverty lies in the poor people's access to credit funds.

In spite of microfinance organizations for the poor around the world, such as Grameen Bank, it's necessary to introduce more innovative financial products and services to achieve the 2030 Sustainable Development Goals in poverty reduction. One of China's current policies to fight poverty is to "give the poor people a leg up to get them going," which means to provide continued support for a few more years after lifting the impoverished households out of poverty, in a bid to promote their sustained development. However, the author's survey found that most grassroots governments had no sufficient funds for such continued support, leading to the phenomenon of "passive poverty reduction" which lifts people out of poverty by gifting them sheep, pigs or chicken for one time. After the impoverished family get rid of poverty, it would be best to provide them with continued support in the following years in the form of credit funds. It would relieve the government from huge financial burden and help the poor make use of the market mechanism for independent operation and stay out of poverty permanently. In fact, compared with the colossal investment needed to lift the poor families out of poverty, the government funds for poverty reduction would never be enough. It's a must to innovate the financial system, products and services for poverty reduction, so as to ensure the poor people's universal access to financial services.

2.5 Build the Resilience of the Poor Against Risks

Poverty-reduction target 1.5 proposes to "by 2030, build the resilience of the poor and those in vulnerable situations, reduce their exposure and vulnerability to climate-related extreme events and other economic, social and environmental shocks and disasters." Vulnerability could be interpreted from two aspects. First, there's often a large group of people barely above the poverty line. Even a mild risk or shock may easily plunge them into poverty again. Second, the poor people are very vulnerable on their own. Any shock or disaster, including climate change, natural disaster, market price fluctuation, disease or accident, could make it difficult for them to rebuild their lives. While both macro and micro policies and measures could be adopted to mitigate such risks and ameliorate the effects of these shocks, long-term institutional development is absolutely necessary. Below some key aspects are discussed.

2.5.1 *Tackling Climate Change*

As the effects of climate change is increasingly felt around the world, the poor are the ones bearing the brunt of it. In this connection, the target of eradicating extreme poverty through sustainable development has been incorporated into the UN's Sustainable Development Goals. In China, three prefectures (Kashgar, Khotan and Kizilsu Kirghiz) in southern Xinjiang, Liupan Mountain areas and Lyuliang Mountain areas have been in water shortage for a long time. Wuling Mountain areas, Wumeng Mountain areas and the rocky desertification areas in Yunnan, Guangxi and Guizhou are mostly characterized by karst features, with a thin layer of soil, serious soil erosion and acute engineering water shortage despite high rainfall. The poor people in these areas are frequent victims to natural disasters. To enhance the resilience of these poor people against the risks and shocks, it's necessary to explore a path of poverty reduction through ecological conservation, which will take a long time.

2.5.2 *Tackling Economic Risks*

In an era of globalization, both domestic and foreign market price fluctuations affect the poor people. As self-employed entities in the market mechanism, the poor households need to improve their adaptability to the market and their ability to tackle economic risks. As the low price in the international grain market and the surplus of domestic grain reserves bit at the same time in 2015, the government lowered the purchase price of corn for temporary reserve in Liaoning, Jilin and Heilongjiang provinces in northeast China and Inner Mongolia by about 12%. As such, the poverty reduction through industrial development in northeast China suffered a blow. The low price of mutton at the same year added to the blow. In this context, the poverty reduction through industrial development for the poverty-stricken households engaged in the production of bulk agricultural products, such as the "company + cooperative + farmer" model, connects small rural households with market, but fails to resolve the difficulties to sell and increase the value of the agricultural products for the poor families.

2.5.3 *Tackling Disease-Related Risks*

In 2014, 42% of the impoverished rural households were made poor by medical bills. Despite the New Rural Cooperative Medical System (NRCMS), the poverty-stricken families still cannot afford the out-of-pocket medical bill. As a result, they either fall below the poverty line or give up the expensive hospitalized treatment. In this sense, the NRCMS is not a pro-poor system. With the focus on insurances for major diseases, the system couldn't help those poor families unable to cover daily medical bills for chronic diseases. The author's survey showed that cardiovascular and cerebrovascular diseases are the leading disease-related causes of poverty. The most important of early symptoms is high blood pressure. Most of them went to the pharmacy to buy medicines at an annual cost of about RMB 3,000, but such expenses cannot be reimbursed for outpatients. In the absence of timely and effective treatment, the high blood pressure largely evolved into cerebral thrombosis, cerebral infarction, myocardial infarction and other major diseases, which deprived the people the ability to work and plunged the family into long-term poverty. All these facts indicate that the current medical insurance system in China cannot fully satisfy the anti-poverty needs at the new stage. Today, under the guidance of national strategy for targeted poverty reduction, the new policies on poverty reduction by improving health are playing a significant role to help solve the problem.

2.6 Conclusions and Discussions

The UN Sustainable Development Goals set clear goals of human development for all countries in the world by 2030, at the core of which is ending poverty in all its forms. The analysis of the UN's poverty-reduction targets by 2030 could lead to the following conclusions and further discussions.

To begin with, the mandatory poverty-reduction target is to eradicate, by 2030, extreme poverty for all people everywhere, measured as living on less than USD 1.9 a day. The current poverty line in rural China is USD 2.29 day/person and China's poverty-reduction goal is to lift all the people living below the poverty line out of poverty by 2020. This means that China will be able to accomplish the UN's mandatory target for poverty reduction by 2020. Another poverty-reduction target set by the UN is to reduce, by 2030, at least by half the proportion of men, women and children of all ages living in poverty in all its forms according to national definitions. For China's 2020 goal of eradicating poverty in all its forms, poverty is defined as a lack of food, clothes and access to education, basic medical service and housing. It's foreseeable that China will fulfill the UN's poverty-reduction target ahead of schedule.

Second, in accordance with the institutional framework proposed by the United Nations, China needs to define poverty multidimensionally, taking both economic security and social services into account. The definition needs to facilitate the efforts toward the 2021–2030 poverty-reduction goal, fit China's conditions and be conducive to the measure of "poverty in all its forms." It shall consider the level of income (consumption) deemed necessary to meet the basic needs, as well as access to public services to meet the needs for the improvement of basic capabilities. It should be noted that the poverty line of USD 1.9 day/person was set by the World Bank based on the standards of the 15 poorest countries in the world. After 2020, China's per capita GDP will exceed 10,000 US dollars and become a high-income country. The absolute poverty line currently recommended by the World Bank for developing countries is USD 3.1 day/person. As a high-income country, China's income/consumption-based poverty line should be raised accordingly. In addition, the use of clean fuels for life, sanitary toilets and other indicators reflecting living standards emphasized in the SDGs need to be specified as mandatory targets for the poverty-reduction programs between 2021 and 2030.

Third, some long-term systems in the UN's poverty-reduction goals provide guide for China. The social protection system should be improved to deliver more benefits for the poor and perfectly complements with the development-oriented poverty reduction. The system for the use of land and natural resources should be innovated constantly to enable the poor people to share the added value. It's a must to keep innovating the patterns of poverty reduction through asset investments, shifting the focus on increasing the asset income for the poor households to encouraging the combination of more asset accumulation with higher asset income so as to counter risks and vulnerability. There's still much space for innovation in poverty reduction through financial services. It's advisable to innovate the development of financial products and services that could promote regional development in poverty-stricken areas; improve cooperative and mutual-aid financial services for specific groups of people; and adopt "Internet +" technology to innovate credit services for the poor. These financial products (services) and commercial financial products (services) would weave a complete financial service network for different groups, which would make it possible to end the "anti-poor and pro-rich" commercial financial services in the market mechanism and deliver universal financial services to the poor people. In addition, the exploration of poverty reduction through ecological conservation, as a way of eradicating poverty through sustainable development, has a promising prospect.

References

HLP. (2013). A new global partnership: Eradicate poverty and transform economies through sustainable development.

Sen, A. K. (1992). *Inequality re-examined*. New York: Russell Sage Foundation.

Sen, A. (2000). *Development as freedom* (Reprint ed), Anchor Books.

Sen, A. (2001). *Poverty and famines*, The Commercial Press.

UN. (2014). Report of the open working group of the general assembly on Sustainable Development Goals. United Nations General Assembly, A/68/970.

UN. (2014). The road to dignity by 2030: Ending poverty, transforming all lives and protecting the planet. The 69th General Assembly session. A/69/700.

United Nations Research Institute for Social Development (UNRISD). (2010). Combating poverty and inequality: Structural change. In *Social policy and politics.*

UNSTT. (2013). A renewed global partnership for development, UN System Task Team on the Post-2015 UN Development Agenda.

Wang, X. (2017). *The measurement of poverty: Theories and methods*, Social Sciences Academic Press.

World Bank. (2001). *Social protection sector strategy paper: From safety net to Springboard*. USA: Washington D.C.

Chapter 3
Poverty in China and the Challenge of the 2030 Poverty Eradication Targets

In light of the SDG target of ending poverty in all its forms everywhere, this chapter will analyze and assess the situation of poverty in China in an all-round way. China will achieve the SDG poverty-reduction goal by 2020, whether measured against the World Bank's extreme poverty line of USD 1.9 day/person, China's rural poverty line or the multidimensional poverty standard of food, clothing and access to education, basic medical service and housing. In this context, this chapter will also examine the key challenges and problems facing China when it works toward more ambitious poverty-reduction goals between 2021 and 2030.

3.1 China's Poverty Line

A set of clearly defined criteria is an essential precondition for poverty assessment in a country. There are three such criteria in China. The first one is the national rural poverty line. It's developed by the State Council Leading Group Office of Poverty Alleviation and Development and measured by National Bureau of Statistics based on poverty monitoring and sample data. The criterion is mainly used for monitoring and assessing the size of the poor population, their distribution and incidence of poverty in China. The second one is the criterion for rural households to be registered as "poor" (poverty identification), established by the above Office mainly for identifying the poor at the micro level and serving as the necessary tool for targeted poverty-reduction programs and policies. The third is the criteria for delisting rural households from the poor register, defined by the same office to assess the authenticity and reliability of poverty-reduction outcomes (see Table 3.1).

X. Wang and X. Zhang, *Towards 2030 – China's Poverty Alleviation and Global Poverty Governance*, International Research on Poverty Reduction,
https://doi.org/10.1007/978-981-15-6356-0_3

Table 3.1 Criteria for rural poverty reduction, registration and delisting from the poor register

Criteria	Definition	Source
National rural poverty line	Per capita net income of RMB 2,300 per year at 2010 constant prices	The central poverty alleviation and development work conference 2011
Criteria for registered poor households (poverty identification)	The registration of the poor emphasizes the family unit and is based on the national poverty line for the countryside. Apart from the key factor of income, the registration also takes into account housing, education, health, etc.	2014: Registration work plan for poverty alleviation and development
Criteria for rural poverty delisting	The state is committed to ensuring that the impoverished rural population has stable access to adequate food and clothing, compulsory education, and basic medical services and housing ("two no-worries and three guarantees") by 2020	2011: The outline for development-oriented poverty reduction for China's Rural areas (2011–2020) 2015: Decision on winning the fight against poverty
	Delisting is household-based. Registered families would be removed from the poor register if they have a stable annual per capita net income above the national poverty line, and guaranteed access to food, clothing, compulsory education, basic medical service and housing	2016: Opinions on establishing a poverty delisting mechanism

Source By the author

3.1.1 China's Rural Poverty Line

The current national rural poverty line was set at the Central Poverty Alleviation and Development Work Conference in 2011. In line with the goal of building a moderately prosperous society in all respects by 2020 and the new stage of the development-oriented poverty reduction in rural China, the central government lifted the national poverty line to the per capita rural net income of RMB 2,300 per year at 2010 constant prices, up by 92% from the standard of RMB 1,196 in 2009.

Pingping Wang, Director of the Department of Household Surveys of National Bureau of Statistics, interpreted the rural poverty line in the Poverty Monitoring Report of Rural China 2015 as follows. "In 2014, in addition to the guarantee of basic housing, the rural poverty line is set at per capita income of RMB 2,800 a year (as against the 2010 constant prices at RMB 2,300), among which the proportion of actual

Table 3.2 Demand for basic food expenditure of rural residents in China in 1985 and 2014, Unit: RMB

Item		1985	2014
Composite average price[a]	Grain (raw)	0.43	2.48
	Vegetable	0.20	2.96
	Pork	3.44	18.39
	Eggs	2.52	9.53
Basic food needs	Commodity grain 500 g/day	0.288	1.653
	Vegetable 500 g/day	0.098	1.478
	Meat 25 g/day	0.086	0.460
	Egg 0.5 per day	0.088	0.334
	Total	0.560	3.925

[a]The composite average price is a simple average of farmers' selling and purchasing prices in rural household surveys. The conversion coefficient of raw grain to commercial grain is 0.75. The consumption expenditure for 50 g of meat or one egg is calculated based on the consumption expenditure for 25 g of meat and half an egg, assuming that one egg weighs 70 g

Source Household Survey Office of the National Bureau of Statistics (2015b)

food expenditure (Engel coefficient) equaled 53.5%, meaning RMB 4.1 day/person for food consumption. Assuming the daily basic needs for food of 500 g of rice or noodle (commodity grain), 500 g of vegetable, 25 g of meat, and half an egg, it would cost RMB 3.924 based on the composite average price of selling and purchasing products for rural resident. The standard of RMB 4.1 is about 1.05 times as much as the basic needs of RMB 3.92. Therefore, the food expenditure in 2014 could meet the need for calorie and protein required for the healthy living." The new national rural poverty line is USD 2.29 day/person (2011 PPP), 21.8% higher than the World Bank's poverty line of USD 1.9 day/person (actually USD 1.88). See Table 3.2 for details.

3.1.2 Registration Standard for Poor Households in Rural China (Poverty Identification)

The central government launched the strategy of targeted poverty reduction in 2013, shifting from the poverty targeting mechanism with contagious poor areas, poor counties and poor villages as the basic unit to the poverty-reduction strategy for targeted poor people and villages. It requires targeted measures in terms of funding, projects and recipients. Every impoverished household is guaranteed help, every village has designated officials to carry out poverty eradication measures, and goals are met within the defined standards. To this end, the State Council Leading Group Office of Poverty Alleviation and Development organized and implemented the work of registering the rural poor households in 28 provinces, autonomous regions and municipalities (excluding Beijing, Tianjin and Shanghai that are free from poor population living below the national poverty line). The threshold for registering the poor is the national rural poverty line of an annual per capita net income of 2,736 yuan (equivalent to the constant price of RMB 2,300 in 2010). The scale of registration is in principle based on a population of 82.49 million, the number of poor people in rural China at the end of 2013 according to the National Bureau of Statistics. If the provincial-level statistics are larger than the national data, an increase of 10% based on the national data is allowable. In individual cases of a larger gap, an appropriately higher increase is allowed. The specific scale of registration shall be determined by the provincial leading group of development-oriented poverty reduction before being submitted to the State Council Leading Group Office of Poverty Alleviation and Development by the provincial leading group office.

In the top-down scale breakdown from townships to administrative villages, a reference method was introduced due to the lack of poverty monitoring base for statistical sampling. The method takes many factors into consideration, including the distance to the towns, infrastructure, public service, per capita net income of farmers, the incidence of poverty in the previous year, household registered population, among others. In line with these standards and scales, the quota of poverty-stricken population for registration was distributed level-by-level from top to administrative villages. The identification of poor households should be first based on the income, while factoring in housing, education, health and others. The poverty identification is based on the unit of household by means of voluntary application, democratic appraisal, public announcement, and level-by-level review.

It can be seen that in the policy design for poverty registration, the scale breakdown of the poor population is based on income, but the identification of poor households is based on multidimensional poverty criteria, factoring in income, education and housing. It also mirrored the idea of "two no-worries, three guarantees." It could be contributed to two reasons. First, the national rural poverty line is based on income/consumption, but in practice, as the farmer's income mainly comes from agribusiness and migrant work (typically informal employment without accurate record of wages and taxation), it's difficult to know their actual income. Second, the *Outline for Development-Oriented Poverty Reduction for China's Rural Areas (2011–2020)* defined multidimensional indictors for poverty-reduction goal as "two no-worries and three guarantees."

3.1.3 Poverty Delisting Criteria in Rural Areas

The poverty-reduction goal as defined in the *Outline for Development-Oriented Poverty Reduction for China's Rural Areas (2011–2020)* (hereinafter referred to as "the Outline" in brief) is that "by 2020, the rural poor people would not worry about food and clothing and would have guaranteed access to compulsory education, basic medical services, and housing" ("two no-worries and three guarantees"). The *Decision on Winning the Fight against Poverty* (hereinafter referred to as "the Decision") issued by the CPC Central Committee and the State Council jointly in December 2015 defined the poverty-reduction goal of "ensuring, by 2020, that the impoverished rural population has stable access to adequate food and clothing, compulsory education, basic medical services, and safe housing." The statement of the "two no-worries and three guarantees" in the Decision is slightly different from that in the Outline, changing from the wording of "housing" to "safe housing." The change gave more priority to ensuring the housing safety for the rural poor population and made safety the primary concern of housing, instead of building cottages or any type of luxury houses.

In the *Opinions on Establishing a Poverty Delisting Mechanism* issued by the central government in April 2016, it's clearly stated that "the poverty delisting mechanism is household-based. The main criterion for removing registered families from the poor register is that they have a stable annual per capita net income above the national poverty line, and have adequate food and clothing and guaranteed access to compulsory education, basic medical service and housing." The document ended the discrepancy surrounding poverty delisting criteria between different places. Previously, there had been three options: national rural poverty line, criteria for registration of rural poor households and national poverty-reduction goal. In areas where poverty was measured by the national rural poverty line, the households with the per capita net income of RMB 2,300 per year (in 2010 constant prices) would be removed from the poor register. In areas where the poverty-reduction goal of "two no-worries and three guarantees" was used as the criteria, the households with adequate food and clothing and guaranteed access to compulsory education, basic medical service and housing would be delisted. The criteria for registration of rural poor households (poverty identification) were a combination of the above two. When the breakdown of the poor population (the first step of the registration process) was concerned, the income-based national rural poverty line was used. When identifying specific rural households living in poverty, multidimensional poverty criteria (income-based, with consideration given to housing, education, health and other factors) were adopted. The Opinions, which emphasizes the multidimensionality of poverty, marks a significant step forward in China's poverty-reduction theory and practice.

China's poverty delisting criteria correspond to the two UN targets for poverty reduction (targets 1.1 and 1.2). Chinese government has made it clear that by 2020, the people removed from the poor register will have a per capita income that is sustainably above the national poverty line, and that they will have adequate food and clothing and guaranteed access to compulsory education, basic medical service and housing. While the income standard corresponds to the UN target 1.1, the other components of the poverty delisting criteria correspond to the UN target 1.2. The criteria may also be seen as the Chinese definition of "poverty in all its forms."

Table 3.3 Poverty in rural China

Year	Poverty line at constant prices of the year (RMB, annual per capita income)	Incidence of poverty (%)	Poor population
1978	366	97	577,039
1980	403	96	276,542
1985	482	78	366,101
1990	807	73	565,849
1995	1,511	60	555,463
2000	1,528	49	846,224
2005	1,742	30	228,662
2010	2,300	17	216,567
2011	2,536	12	712,238
2012	2,625	10	29,899
2013	2,736	8	58,249
2014	2,800	7	27,017
2015	2,855	5	75,575

Note The data in the above table is based on the 2015 standard, the new rural poverty line at 2011 constant prices. The data for the years from 1978 to 2010 is converted in line with the 2015 standard
Source The data from 1978 to 2010 comes from China Rural Poverty Monitoring Report 2015 by the Household Survey Office of the National Bureau of Statistics. The data from 2011 to 2015 comes from Statistical Communiqué of the People's Republic of China on the 2015 National Economic and Social Development

3.2 Poverty in China Today

3.2.1 Income/Consumption-Based Poverty

In line with China's rural poverty line of RMB 2,300 (in 2010 constant prices) for the annual per capita income, the rural poor population was 55.75 million in 2015, with the incidence of poverty at 5.7%. Since 1978, over 700 million rural people have been lifted out of poverty (see Table 3.3). Measured against the current rural poverty line, the incidence of poverty in China has been quite low, but due to a large population, there are still 55.75 million people in poverty.

In 1981, China had a poor population of 878 million, with the incidence of poverty at 88.32%, accounting for 43.95% of the global poor population. Measured against the World Bank's poverty line of USD 1.9 per person per day, the poor population in China dropped to 57 million in 2015,[1] the incidence of poverty fell to 4.2%, while the share of global poor population dropped to 8.18%. There's no doubt that China

[1] It's forecasted by the UNDP in evaluating the progress toward the attainment of MDGs. According to the statistics released by the UNDP in October 2016, measured against the poverty line of USD 1.9 per person per day, the incidence of poverty in urban and rural China stood at 1.85% in 2013, with a poor population of 25.11 million, far below the previous forecast.

Table 3.4 Poverty in China and the world (the poverty line of USD 1.9 per day)

Year	Poor population (million)			Incidence of poverty (%)	
	World	China	Proportion	World	China
1981	1,997.28	877.80	43.95	44.30	88.32
1984	1,955.26	785.40	40.17	41.16	75.75
1987	1,864.55	659.53	35.37	37.25	60.84
1990	1,958.57	755.81	38.59	37.10	66.58
1993	1,916.70	671.71	35.05	34.65	57.00
1996	1,715.79	511.98	29.84	29.69	42.05
1999	1,751.45	507.86	29.00	29.08	40.54
2002	1,645.12	409.09	24.87	26.29	31.95
2005	1,401.01	244.45	17.45	21.59	18.75
2008	1,253.90	194.06	15.48	18.65	14.65
2010	1,119.75	149.56	13.36	16.27	11.18
2011	983.33	106.19	10.80	14.12	7.90
2012	896.70	87.39	9.75	12.73	6.47
2015	702.00	57.00	8.18	9.60	4.20

Source World Bank—PovcalNet, accessed on March 22, 2016. The 2015 data is the forecast of World Bank

has made remarkable achievements in poverty reduction (see Table 3.4). Excluding China's contribution, there would be an increase of poor population in the world between 1981 and 2002.

3.2.2 *Multidimensional Poverty*

Measured against the global multidimensional poverty index, the incidence of multidimensional poverty in China was 4.0% in 2014 and the population in multidimensional poverty was 55.27 million. In June 2017, Oxford Poverty & Human Development Initiative (OPHI) launched the 2017 Global MPI, covering 103 countries that are home to 76% of the world's population, or 5.4 billion people. Of this proportion, 26.5% of people (1.45 billion) are identified as multidimensionally poor, among whom 48% live in South Asia and 36% in sub-Saharan Africa. A proportion of 72% of MPI poor people live in middle-income countries. The global MPI measures poverty across three dimensions and 10 indicators: health (nutrition and mortality), education (years of schooling, school attendance) and living standards (cooking fuel, sanitation, drinking water, electricity, housing, assets). It captures the deprivations facing the households, the average number of the deprived poor people and the severity of deprivations facing the poor families.

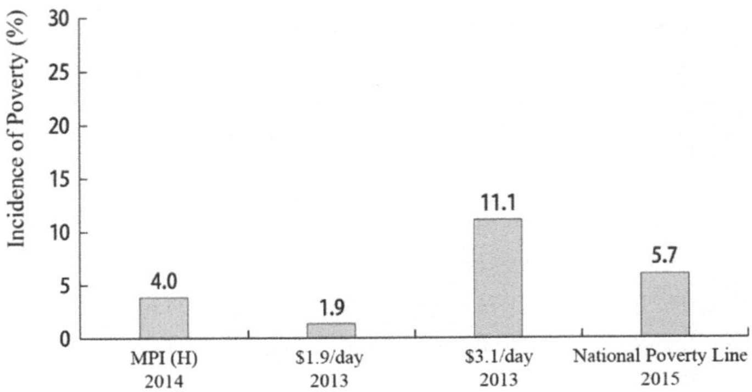

Fig. 3.1 Multidimensional poverty and income-based poverty in China (based on different criteria). *Note* The national poverty line refers to the farmers' per capita net income of RMB 2,300 at 2010 constant prices. The incidence of poverty only covers rural areas, excluding urban areas. *Source* MPI data comes from OPHI, the data of USD 1.9 and USD 3.1 from the World Bank, and the national poverty line from National Bureau of Statistics of China

In 2014, China's MPI (k = 33.3%) was 0.017, the multidimensional headcount ratio was 4.0%, the multidimensional poverty intensity was 41.3% and the MPI poor population was 55.27 million. When the dimensional poverty threshold "k" ranges between 20 and 33.3%, the vulnerable people in China comprised 16.8% in 2014, which means that 16.8% of Chinese people might be identified as MPI poor (k = 33.3%). The people in severe poverty (k = 50%) made up 0.3%, or 4.1 million Chinese in severe poverty in 2014. Measured against the MPI indicators, more than half of these people are MPI poor. Figure 3.1 shows that China progressed better in the MPI poverty reduction than in the income-based poverty reduction. This might be contributed to China's multidimensional definition of poverty. The poverty reduction work in China involves more than 40 departments and the relating policy system is a combination of multidimensional development-oriented poverty reduction with the guarantee of social securities.

China's MPI poor population is mainly distributed in rural areas, central and western regions. In 2014, the incidence of multidimensional poverty in urban China was 1.9% and that in rural China was 6.7%. Unlike other developing countries, the incidence of poverty in urban China has been low all the time, which also explains why China's national poverty-reduction strategy (the Outline) has targeted merely at the rural poverty. In terms of regional distribution, the incidence of multidimensional poverty in eastern, central and western areas was 1.9, 3.2 and 8.1%, respectively.

China performs the worst in terms of three indicators: nutrition, years of schooling and cooking fuel. Judging from the contribution of 10 indicators to MPI, the top three indicators in China in 2014 were nutrition (33.4%), schooling years (16.4%) and cooking fuel (11.2%). As for nutrition and schooling years, long-term efforts would surely lead to significant progress in poverty reduction.

3.3 Challenges of Eradicating Poverty by 2030

By 2020, China will be able to eradicate extreme poverty, measured as people living on less than USD 1.9 a day, which is also the poverty-reduction target 1.1 of the Sustainable Development Goal. In line with China's income-based poverty line and the multidimensional poverty delisting criteria of "two no-worries and three guarantees," China will also eradicate "poverty in all its forms" by 2020, which is the poverty-reduction target 1.2 of the Sustainable Development Goal. Therefore, the following part shall be dedicated to the discussions about China's main challenges toward a higher level of poverty reduction between 2021 and 2030.

3.3.1 Alleviating Regional Relative Poverty

In 2015, half of 55.75 million poor Chinese lived in 14 contiguous poverty-stricken areas, including the rocky desertification areas in Yunnan, Guangxi and Guizhou, Wuling Mountain areas, Wumeng Mountain areas, Qinling-Daba Mountains areas and Dabie Mountain areas, all home to no less than 3 million poor people. In addition to a large poor population, these contiguous areas feature tough natural conditions, few arable land and key national eco-function zones. These areas are much less developed in economy compared with the eastern China, with infrastructure, public service and technology below the national average. The regional economic growth, due to the lack in driving force, can contribute little to poverty reduction.

First, these areas feature unfavorable geological location, backward infrastructure and public services, as well as poor environment and conditions for development. Mainly perched in the transitional zones between the first, second and third tiers of the terrain in China, these contiguous poverty-stricken areas are mostly at the marginal areas of provinces, autonomous regions and municipalities, far away from the downtown, with little radiation effect and driving force for growth. Among 832 poor counties in contiguous areas and key poor counties, 359 counties are located in restricted development zones and nearly half of these towns have no access to highways of grade II and above.

Second, these areas feature special poverty. First, in the Karst areas in the rocky desertification areas in Yunnan, Guangxi and Guizhou, Wuling Mountain areas, and Wumeng Mountain areas, the prominent problem lies in the lack of land, afflicting 10 million poor people. Second, in the four prefectures (Kashgar, Khotan, Kizilsu Kirghiz and Akesu) in southern Xinjiang, the problem of water shortage and drought affected nearly 1 million poor people. Third, in the Qinghai-Tibet Plateau, Tibet and Tibetan areas in Qinghai, Sichuan, Yunnan and Gansu provinces, the lack of oxygen and low temperature affected about 1.4 million poor people. Fourth, on the Loess Plateau, including Liupan Mountain area and Lyuliang Mountain area, some 3.4 million poor people suffer from drought and water shortage. Fifth, in areas with high incidence of endemic diseases, the Kaschin-Beck disease struck 131 counties and incapacitated some patients in their 40 s. Sixth, among 136 land border counties, 72 are impoverished and the mountainous areas along the western Yunnan border are home to nearly 2 million poor people.

Regional poverty in China takes special forms with interwoven features of fragile eco-environment, poor infrastructure and public services, as well as a large poor population. By 2020, the battle against poverty over the 13th Five-Year Plan period (2016–2020) will end regional poverty overall and fulfill the poverty-reduction target of "two no-worries and three guarantees." Relatively speaking, however, a majority of these regions will still be in relative poverty. In this connection, the Chinese government needs to identify and reduce poverty after 2020 based on an overall consideration for regional development, ecological conservation and narrower development gap. This will continue to be a major challenge facing China's poverty reduction between 2021 and 2030.

As China ushers in a new stage (2021–2030) of poverty reduction, is it necessary to re-identify regional poverty? By 2020, 592 key counties for national development-oriented poverty reduction work will all be lifted out of poverty. Is it necessary to identify a new batch of "socioeconomically weak counties" so that they could get continuous support to narrow the regional development gap? In the author's opinion, lifting the above-mentioned 592 key counties out of poverty signifies the massive eradication of regional extreme poverty, which marks a significant milestone in China's anti-poverty history. Given the long-term goal of common prosperity for everyone, China still needs to identify the "socioeconomically weak counties" to continue with development-oriented poverty reduction work in regions affected by relative poverty. The combination of poverty reduction oriented toward regional development with that targeting villages and households will surely lead to more remarkable achievements in poverty reduction.

3.3.2 Development of the Vulnerable People

The vulnerable or marginal population refers to the relatively poor people living above the extreme poverty line but below a higher poverty standard. They are not in extreme poverty, but their life is still unstable and they are highly likely to fall into poverty again due to their vulnerability to risks. The following part will assess the vulnerable population in China from the perspectives of income-based poverty and multidimensional poverty.

1. Income-based vulnerable population

This chapter defines the people living on between USD 1.9 and USD 3.1 a day as vulnerable people. In this connection, Fig. 3.2 shows the vulnerable population in China. Measured against the World Bank's extreme poverty line of USD 1.9 a day, less than 1% of Chinese people were in extreme poverty in 2015. Given that China is a middle- and high-income country, measured against the poverty line of USD 3.1

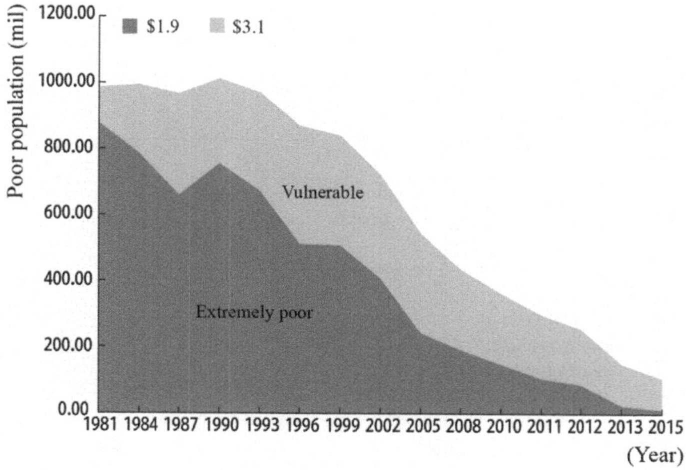

Fig. 3.2 Extreme poverty and vulnerable people in China. *Note* The size of China's poor population living on less than USD 3.1 a day is forecasted by the author. *Source* World Bank: PovcalNet, accessed on July 15, 2016

a day for middle-income countries, there were 151 million poor Chinese in 2013, including 126 million in rural areas and 24.83 million in urban areas, registering an incidence of poverty of 11.09%.[2] The author predicted that there were roughly 107 million people living on less than USD 3.1 a day in 2015. If we define the people living on between USD 1.9 and USD 3.1 a day as the vulnerable population above the extreme poverty line, the population was about 100 million. By 2020, extreme poverty will be eliminated and a moderately prosperous society in all respects will be built in China. A majority of some 100 million people currently living on less than USD 3.1 a day will become a part of the vulnerable population above the extreme poverty line between 2021 and 2030. This group will be the focus in the new stage of fighting relative poverty after 2020.

2. MPI-based vulnerable population

Based on the definition of global MPI, we define the population corresponding to the multidimensional poverty threshold "k" at 33.3% as the MPI poor people, and the population corresponding to "k" between 20 and 33% as the vulnerable people. In 2014, the MPI poor population was about 50 million and the vulnerable population was roughly 230 million in China. In spite of large-scale and multidimensional targeted poverty reduction work in China, the top indicators contributing to MPI poverty, including nutrition and schooling years, still require long-term efforts. The other top indicator "cooking fuel" is not included in China's goal for the fight against poverty. Under the influence of these three key indicators, it can be predicted that

[2]Data source: World Bank: PovcalNet, accessed on August 9, 2017.

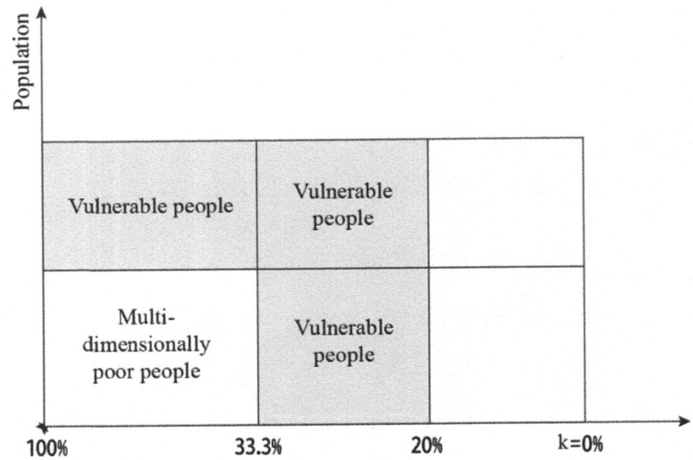

Fig. 3.3 China's multidimensionally vulnerable population

the multidimensionally vulnerable population in China should be no less than 100 million in 2021 (see Fig. 3.3).

These are a preliminary estimate of a relatively poor group above China's extreme MPI poverty line based on assessment of 10 indicators across three dimensions: education, health and living standards. With the elimination of extreme multidimensional poverty, the majority of the vulnerable people will become the focus for China's development-oriented poverty reduction after 2020. The size of this group needs to be estimated based on the new standard for multidimensional poverty and population data.

3.3.3 Narrower Income Gap

Both Fig. 3.4 and Table 3.5 indicate a large income gap among Chinese residents. Despite the year-by-year declining Gini coefficient of Chinese residents' income from the peak at 0.491, it's still as high as 0.462 in 2015, beyond the income gap recognized across the world. A larger Gini coefficient will make the economic growth less pro-poor, which will further damage the fairness of opportunities and make the economic growth less inclusive. The long-term goal of the CPC is to build a society of common prosperity for everyone, which requires a small income gap. Therefore, between 2021 and 2030, one of the challenges facing the poverty reduction in China is to effectively narrow the income gap and development gap, which is a main anti-poverty goal in the stage of fighting relative poverty after 2020.

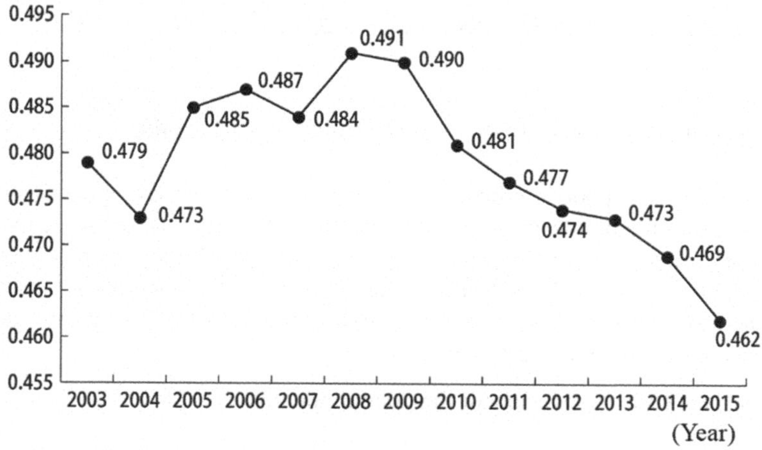

Fig. 3.4 Gini coefficient of per capita income of Chinese residents. *Source* The website of National Bureau of Statistics

Table 3.5 Residents' disposable income by quintile in 2015

Regions	Nationwide	Rural	Urban	Urban/Rural
Per capita disposable income (RMB)	21,966	11,422	31,195	2.73
Lowest (20%)	5,221	3,086	12,231	3.96
Low (20%)	11,894	7,221	21,446	2.97
Middle (20%)	19,320	10,311	29,105	2.82
High (20%)	29,438	14,537	38,572	2.65
Highest (20%)	54,544	26,014	65,082	2.50
Highest/lowest	10.45	8.43	5.32	–

Source Household Survey Office of the National Bureau of Statistics (2015a)

The income gap in rural China is even greater. Table 3.5 shows that the ratio of the highest to the lowest quintile is as high as 8.43. The per capita annual disposable income of the lowest quintile (20%) was only RMB 3,086. It means that the income of the lowest quintile (20%) has barely surpassed the national rural poverty line (RMB 2,855 in 2015).

The income inequality made it a must for China to improve the equality in income distribution while striving to increase per capita income of residents. Improving the income distribution will be more effective for poverty reduction. It requires the establishment of more pro-poor social protection system and wealth accumulation system, so as to improve the income distribution in both short and long terms.

3.3.4 Poverty Due to Disease and Incapability Due to Old Age

1. Illness deprives the poor of the working ability and decent life.

At present, 42% of poor households in China are due to severe disease, chronic disease or disability of one or more family members. Poverty due to disease requires more complicated anti-poverty policies and measures, posing greater challenges to poverty reduction. Illness bites the poor households from the following perspectives: direct medical expenses; loss of working ability; the need for family care; dented confidence in self-reliance, just to name a few.

2. Defuse the risks of diseases for the poor population.

China has established the New Rural Cooperative Medical System (NRCMS) to effectively mitigate the risk of serious diseases for the rural residents. However, the current system is not enough to cope with the risk of poverty caused by disease. Take Hunan Province for example. In 2015, there were over 4 million poor people in the province and more than 500,000 households were plunged into poverty by disease. According to the Health Statistics of Hunan Province in 2013, a high proportion of the medical expenses for the poor people occurred in township clinics and county-level hospitals. In 2013, the per capita medical expenses of inpatients were RMB 1,097.6 at township clinics and RMB 6,338.9 at county-level hospitals, as against RMB 11,000 at state-level hospitals (see Fig. 3.5). Such medical expenses alone, excluding the related expenditures for transportation, accommodation and family care, would be a heavy economic burden for the poor households and is likely to result in enduring poverty for years. The medical assistance system for severe diseases has been put in place, but still not enough in coverage and support. In 2016, the National Health Commission and 14 other departments jointly issued the Guidelines on Implementing

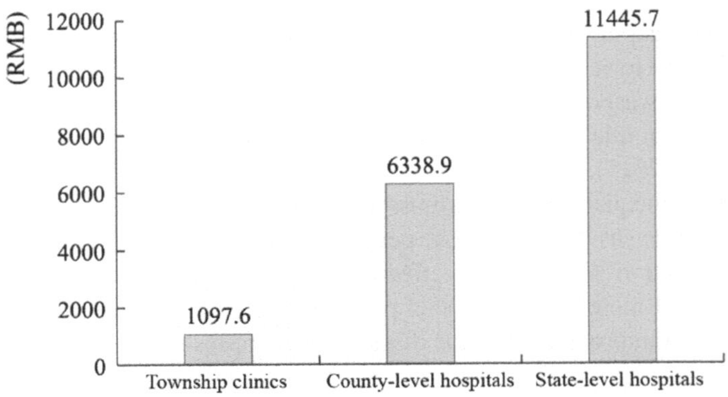

Fig. 3.5 Per capita medical expenses of inpatients in hospitals at various levels in Hunan Province in 2013

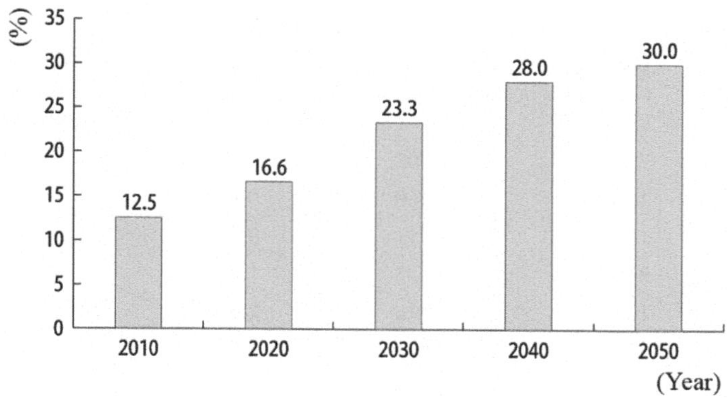

Fig. 3.6 Ratio of people over 60 in China. *Source* Yushao Wu. Ed. *China Report of the Development on Aging Cause (2013)*. Social Sciences Academic Press (China). 2013

Poverty Alleviation Project through Health Promotion to improve the system from various aspects. First, improve the new rural cooperative medical insurance to effectively relieve the burden of medical expenses for the poor rural residents. Second, increase severe disease assistance. Third, put in place the supplementary commercial insurance system for serious diseases. Fourth, provide classified treatment for serious diseases and chronic diseases. All these measures are being implemented.

3. The emerging old-age poverty requires institutional countermeasures

China has become an aging society and will see further increase in the proportion of the elderly poor between 2021 and 2030. A striking feature associated with aging is the incapability of the elderly population. The extra cost of living and relative cost for elders living alone and incapable elders at advanced age will be much higher.[3] According to the UN 2015 report, the largest low-fertility countries are China, the United States, Brazil, Russia and Japan.[4] As a result of low fertility and high life expectancy, China will become a highly aging society by 2030. According to the forecast of the China National Committee on Aging, the proportion of people over the age of 60 in China will reach 23.3% by 2030 (see Fig. 3.6). Experts opined that the launch of the two-child policy will help address the aging issue to a certain extent, but it won't stop China from entering the aging society. The urbanization and population mobility came with a large number of "empty nests" and "left-behind elders" in rural China, especially the impoverished rural areas. The poverty-stricken villages have seen an increasing number of disabled senior citizens due to aging, diseases and disabilities, posing serious challenges to the strategies and policies relating to development-oriented poverty reduction implemented since 1986. It's imperative for China to explore innovative poverty-reduction models, strategies and policies that befit the era of aging society and urbanization.

[3]Xu and Wang et al. (2011).

[4]United Nations Department of Economic and Social Affairs/Population Division (2015).

Table 3.6 Poverty and landholding in rural Bangladesh (1978–1979)

Landholding class (acres of land owned)	Percentage of total households in class (%)	Mean income (Taka/month)	Mean landholdings (acres)	Headcount index (percentage of population)
Landless	7.1	508	0	93
0–0.5	36.1	560	0.1	93
0.5–1.0	10.5	711	0.7	84
1.0–1.5	8.9	783	1.2	78
1.5–2.5	12.1	912	2.0	68
2.5–5.0	13.8	1,613	3.5	45
5.0–7.5	5.7	1,516	6.0	23
7.5+	5.8	2,155	14.0	10
Total	100	865	2.1	70

Source World Bank (1990)

3.3.5 *Lack of Assets and Economic Resources*

A very natural feature of poverty is its association with the lack in the ownership of and right to use the productive assets. The lack of asset breeds poverty, and vice versa. In other words, the lack of assets is closely interrelated with poverty.[5] Of particular concern are the farmers who lost their lands in the process of urbanization and the migrant people's lack of assets and right to economic resources.

1. Land is the productive asset that's most closely related to poverty

In South Asia, most of the poor are landless workers. Until today, India and Bangladesh have a large poor population and high incidence of poverty. India continues to be home to the largest population in extreme poverty. In South Asia, poverty is closely associated with the fact that the farmers have no right for land ownership. Similarly, in sub-Saharan Africa, the majority of the poor are small household farmers or pastoralists. According to an earlier study report by the World Bank, 43.2% of rural households in Bangladesh have no land or less than 0.5 acres of land, with the incidence of poverty among them as high as 93%, compared to merely 10% among the farmers with 14 acres of land per household (see Table 3.6).

2. Land system is a "double-edged sword" for poverty reduction

China's success in the large-scale elimination of extreme poverty is closely related to the household contracting system of rural land that was launched in the 1980s. The system endowed the farmers with the landholding right (long-term use) in a fair manner. Figure 3.7 shows that in 1959 and 1960 when the collective ownership of rural land dominated and the farmers were forced to cooperate, the total factor

[5]Ray (2002).

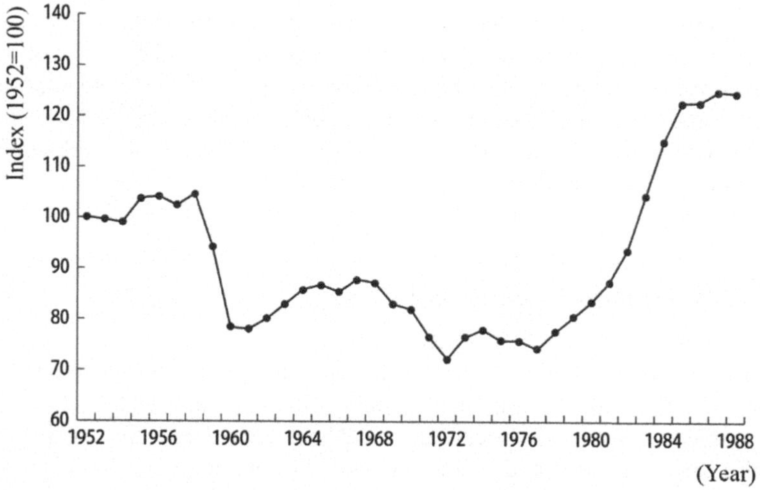

Fig. 3.7 China's agricultural total factor productivity index (1952–1988). *Source* Justin Yifu Lin. *Institution, Technology and Agricultural Development in China.* Shanghai Sanlian Bookstore, Shanghai People's Publishing House. 1994:16–43

productivity of agriculture plummeted and maintained that way for a long term till the reform in 1978. After the household contracting system of rural land was implemented in 1978, the total factor productivity increased rapidly.[6] Between 1981 and 1990, the population in extreme poverty, measured as people living on less than USD 1.25 a day, dropped by 148 million, which went some way toward explaining the significance of land system and asset rights to the elimination of extreme poverty.

It brings us to the next point: the urbanization rate in China will keep increasing between 2021 and 2030. In this process, land will become a double-edged sword that could either lift people out of poverty or plunge people into poverty. Some suburban farmers got rid of poverty, thanks to the compensation for their land expropriated, and a few even got rich overnight and became owners of several homes. But land expropriation could also throw some farmers into poverty: their income increased slightly in the short term, but their living standards lowered in the long term. In line with the current definition, the land-lost farmers refer to a per capita cultivated land of less than 0.05 *mu* in a rural family whose land was expropriated in accordance with the law. There's no official statistics on the number of land-lost farmers in China. Researcher Yansui Liu from the Institute of Geographic Sciences and Natural Resources Research, Chinese Academy of Social Sciences, pointed out at a forum that there were 112 million land-lost farmers in China by the end of 2014.

During the period from 2021 to 2030, China needs to conduct in-depth and meticulous investigations into land-lost farmers and other economic resources that are vital to poverty reduction, for the purpose of working out some pro-poor institutional arrangements relating to asset rights. In the next stage, how to make inclusive

[6]Lin (1994).

and pro-poor institutional arrangements concerning economic rights will be a major challenge facing China's sustainable poverty reduction. It will be of great importance to prevent the intergenerational transmission of poverty, and more importantly, the achievement of China's long-term goal for common prosperity for everyone. It's also the key to translating the CPC Central Committee's vision of development for "shared benefits" into practice.

3.3.6 The Human Capital Gap

Investment in people to build a higher level of human capital is the linchpin to human development. The building of human capital involves the fairness and effectiveness of basic public services, such as education and healthcare. Given the existing degree of unfairness in education and health, this would be another great challenge facing China's sustainable poverty reduction and narrower development gap between 2021 and 2030.

1. Intergenerational transmission of poverty due to unfair allocation of educational resources

Early childhood education for children aged 0–3 and preschool education for those aged 4–6 are two key educational stages for human capital development, featuring considerable urban–rural and regional inequalities in China. There is a huge gap between urban and rural areas in the allocation of early childhood educational resources. Nearly 100% of the four- to six-year-olds in the cities go to the kindergartens, and that proportion is only 30% in rural areas and even lower in poor rural areas. In the "Guidelines on Accelerating the Development of Education in the Central and Western China" issued by the General Office of the State Council in 2016, China sets the goal of increasing the three-year preschool gross enrollment rate in the central and western China to 70% by 2020. Assuming the fulfillment of this goal as scheduled, there will still be 30% of eligible children without access to the three-year preschool education in these areas. The development-oriented poverty reduction has long focused more on improving productivity and increasing income of the people with the ability to work. The human capital development has long focused more on vocational education and skill training. The importance of preschool education for the fight against poverty has long been neglected. In future, China needs to be more aware of the importance of investing in people, especially children, and in the future, while making "elimination of poverty among children in all its dimensions" a key component of anti-poverty strategy. The State Council Leading Group Office of Poverty Alleviation and Development could play its role in the overall cross-departmental allocation of resources to establish a highly effective institutional framework to end poverty among children. The author is confident that this would effectively disrupt the intergenerational transmission of poverty.

2. Intergenerational transmission of poverty due to the lack in maternal and child healthcare and early childhood nutrition improvement schemes

China has made extraordinary achievements in maternal and child healthcare. In a few contiguous poor areas, however, the maternal and child healthcare measured against key development indicators is still quite backward. In 2013, the under-five mortality rate, infant mortality rate and neonatal mortality rate in rural areas were, respectively, 2.4, 2.2 and 2 times as high as that in cities. Except in some individual provinces and regions, a higher child and maternal mortality rate is typically associated with the lower per capita GDP in the provinces or regions. In coastal developed areas, such as Shanghai, Jiangsu and Zhejiang, the maternal mortality rate is below 4/100,000 and the perinatal mortality rate is below 5‰, which has basically reached the level of developed countries. In poor areas, such as Xinjiang, Qinghai and Gansu, the maternal mortality rate fluctuates between 24/100,000 and 36/100,000 and the perinatal mortality rate is above 8‰. In Tibet, the perinatal and maternal mortality rate is as high as 24.04‰ and 176/100,000, respectively.[7]

3.4 Conclusions and Discussions

This chapter leads us to the following conclusions and extended discussions.

By 2020, China can achieve the goal of eradicating extreme poverty, measured as people living on less than USD 1.9 per person per day, and the goal of "ending poverty in all its forms" to ensure adequate food and clothing and guaranteed access to education, basic medical service and housing for the poor as defined by the multidimensional poverty standard. While formulating the outline for poverty reduction over the next decade from 2021 to 2030, China needs to consider the following questions.

1. In the special contiguous poverty-stricken areas, how to address intertwined contributors to poverty by improving infrastructure, public services and ecology, while creating a fairer environment for the targeted poverty reduction of the poor and the sustainable development of the impoverished areas? After 2020, China needs to define regional poverty and focus on the elimination of relative regional poverty.
2. How to establish a multidimensional poverty standard more suitable for China's conditions, with a view to increasing the income of the poor and the vulnerable, improving their capability for development, and ultimately achieving substantial improvement in the living standards of the poor?
3. How to translate the CPC Central Committee's vision of development for "shared benefits" into practice, put in place more pro-poor property right system and other economic systems, and continue to narrow development gap in the process of urbanization, so as to better benefit the poor? China should pay special attention

[7]Ma (2016).

to the land-lost farmers in the process of urbanization and the lack of assets and rights to economic resources for the migrant people.

4. How to improve the relevant systems such as for education, medical care, assistance and old-age care, to deliver more inclusive and pro-poor systems vital to human development that cover all vulnerable groups of children, women, the elderly and the disabled? While increasing investment in children and in the future, China should strive to address the relative poverty of migrant population and left-behind elderly amid the course of urbanization and aging society.

References

Household Survey Office of the National Bureau of Statistics. (2015a). China Yearbook of Household Survey 2016, China Statistics Press.

Household Survey Office of the National Bureau of Statistics. (2015b). China Rural Poverty Monitoring Report 2015, China Statistics Press.

Lin, J. Y. (1994). *Institution, technology and agricultural development in China* (pp. 16–43). Shanghai Sanlian Bookstore, Shanghai People's Publishing House.

Ma, X. (2016). Proposal on Improving the Maternal and Child Healthcare Services in Poor Areas. Proposal No. 0128 at the Third Session of the 12th National Committee of the Chinese People's Political Consultative Conference, Chinese People's Political Consultative Conference Media Network.

National Bureau of Statistics. (2016). Statistical Communiqué of the People's Republic of China on the 2015 National Economic and Social Development. Official website of National Bureau of Statistics.

Ray, D. (2002). *Development economics* (Vol. 241), Peking University Press.

United Nations Department of Economic and Social Affairs/Population Division. (2015). World population prospects: The 2015 revision, Key findings and advance tables. New York: United Nations.

World Bank. (1990). *World development report* (Vol. 32).

Xu, L., & Wang, X., et al. (2011) Estimation of the relative cost of disability of the Elderly in China. *Chinese Journal of Population Science, 2*.

Chapter 4
Development-Oriented Poverty Reduction: A System with Chinese Characteristics

China has since 1986 begun to explore ways for massive elimination of extreme poverty. With more than three decades of hard work, China has devised a distinct system of development-oriented poverty alleviation. The system incorporates a definition of poverty from multiple dimensions based on Chinese culture, dedicated and cross-sector government agencies of poverty reduction at national and local levels, specific poverty-reduction strategies and policies in support of such strategies. The system is mainly characterized by commitment to the reform and opening-up to foster pro-poor growth, the government-led special programs in development-oriented poverty reduction, the development-oriented poverty alleviation to improve the poor people's capabilities for self-reliance, the mobilization of all social sectors to form a synergy for pro-poor development and the pro-poor social protection system. This chapter briefly interprets the development-oriented poverty alleviation system with Chinese characteristics, covering the multidimensional definition of "poverty" in Chinese, the organization of state institutions for poverty reduction, the assessment of China's poverty-reduction strategy and a review of the current targeted poverty alleviation strategy.

4.1 Multidimensionality of the Definition of "Poverty"

Eliminating or reducing poverty is a basic requirement for the development of human society. The definition and understanding of poverty in a culture are crucial to the national strategies and policies on poverty reduction. In traditional Chinese culture, development means that "a competent provision was secured for the aged till their death, employment for the able-bodied, and the means of growing up to the young. Kindness and compassion are offered to widows, orphans, childless men, and those who were disabled by disease, so that they were all sufficiently maintained," as defined in the *Book of Rites*. The Chinese equivalent of "poverty" is *pin-kun* (贫困).

X. Wang and X. Zhang, *Towards 2030 – China's Poverty Alleviation and Global Poverty Governance*, International Research on Poverty Reduction,
https://doi.org/10.1007/978-981-15-6356-0_4

Fig. 4.1 Definition of poverty

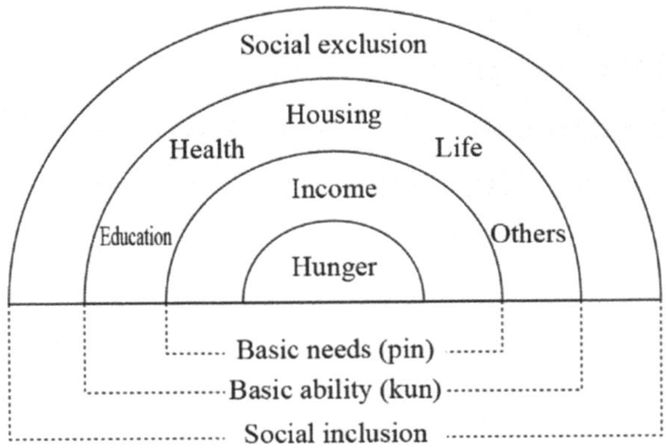

The *Shuowen Jiezi* (literally meaning "explaining graphs and analyzing characters"), a Chinese dictionary from the Han Dynasty, defines *pin* as "few assets." The *Xinhua Dictionary* defines it as "less income and difficult life" and *kun* as "a state of being trapped in hardships or a situation that's difficult to get rid of." Therefore, we can say that *pin–kun* mainly refers to a state of being trapped in hardships or a situation that's difficult to get rid of due to meagre income or asset, including the hardships relating to food, clothing, housing, traveling, education, health and environment. *Pin* and *kun* are interactional. *Pin* makes it impossible to go to school, see a doctor or improve living conditions due to the lack in money, leading to *kun*. On the other hand, *kun* makes it impossible to get education and healthcare, and thus no way to form human capital and physical capital, which in turn exacerbates *pin*, leading to the "poverty trap."[1]

Figure 4.1 shows a framework for the definition of poverty. The first layer of poverty is hunger, the core of poverty. The second layer refers to the insufficient income to meet the basic needs of individuals or families, which is the basic meaning of the word "poverty" in English. The third layer relates to the acquisition of basic capabilities involving education, health, housing and daily necessities (such as durable consumer goods), corresponding to the multidimensional poverty in English. Such extended understanding of poverty is based on Amartya Sen's study on poverty and welfare economics, which corresponds to *kun* in Chinese. Therefore, the definition of *pin–kun* in Chinese covers both the basic needs and the basic capabilities, which is multidimensional. Furthermore, there is a fourth layer of poverty: social exclusion. It pays more attention to social integration between different races and different communities. Generally speaking, the developed countries attach higher importance to social inclusion.

In this sense, the definition of *pin–kun* incorporates *pin* caused by insufficient income, as well as *kun* of individuals and families in unfavorable natural and social environment. This explains the major difference in connotations of *pin–kun* in Chinse

[1] Wang (2012).

and poverty in English, which plays a decisive role in the organization of state institutions and path for development-oriented poverty reduction with Chinese characteristics. Helping the poor and doing good has long been a traditional virtue in China. Chinese government's definition of *pin–kun* has been evolving with the socioeconomic development. According to the *Notice on Promoting Economic Development in Impoverished Areas* issued by the State Council in 1987, the poor population refers to the people in absolute poverty who suffer great difficulties in material subsistence (insufficient food and clothing, no housing) and can only maintain shrinking or simple reproduction. This definition is based on the basic needs, reflecting the core of *pin*. *The Opinions on Establishing a Poverty Delisting Mechanism* made it clear in 2015 that Chinese government's goal to eliminate poverty is multidimensional, that is, by 2020, to achieve the goal of poverty reduction so that those who have been living in poverty no longer have to worry about food and clothing, with guaranteed access to compulsory education, basic medical treatment and housing security. The new goal takes into account both basic needs and basic capabilities, both *pin* and *kun*. Compared with the 1987 definition, it extends to include "education and health" for the basic capabilities, in addition to basic needs for food, clothing and housing.

China has long been implementing the multidimensional development-oriented poverty-reduction policies. Based on the large-scale development of infrastructure and public services, the development-oriented poverty-alleviation model was adopted to improve the overall environment for the development of poverty-stricken areas and the poor people's capabilities for development. By virtue of systems on land, labor, agricultural products market, population mobility and others, the poor will be given the right to freely produce, work, exchange and move, and thus resolve the development difficulties for the poor. Income-support policies will be introduced to achieve the poverty-reduction goal, and social policies and interventions to help the poor get out of the predicament, improve their capabilities for development and enhance the social inclusiveness and mobility. China's multidimensional development-oriented poverty-reduction policies were carried out by cross-sector state institutions, a key takeaway for other developing countries.

4.2 Establishing Special Government Agencies that Transcend Ministerial Divisions

In 1979, the central government proposed to set up a special committee in the State Council, comprising heads of relevant departments for coordinative planning and organization. From the aspects of finance, materials and technologies, the poverty-stricken areas in northwestern and southwestern China, some former revolutionary base areas, remote mountainous areas, ethnic minority areas and border areas shall be prioritized for support in production, in a bid to get rid of poverty. To this end, two special institutions were set up. One is the State Council Leading Group of Agricultural Development in Three Western Areas[2] established in 1982. The other is the State Council Leading Group of Economic Development in Poor Areas established in 1986, which was renamed the State Council Leading Group of Poverty Alleviation and Development in 1993.

In 1982, the State Council decided to form the Leading Group of Agricultural Development in Three Western Areas, comprising the heads from a dozen of state institutions, such as Ministry of Agriculture, State Economic Commission, Ministry of Water and Power, Ministry of Finance, Ministry of Forestry, Ministry of Commerce, Ministry of Civil Affairs, State Science and Technology Commission, Chinese Academy of Sciences and State Planning Commission. An office was set up for this purpose, namely Three Western Areas Office in short, mainly responsible for convening various sectors, formulating construction plans and using special funds to coordinate and resolve key difficulties in agricultural development of the three western areas, to eliminate poverty and prevent ecological deterioration. A decade of hard work has paid off (see Box 4.1).

Box 4.1 Agricultural Development in Three Western Areas

From 1983 to 1992, during the 10-year agricultural construction in Three Western Areas, the central government earmarked RMB 200 million each year for water conservancy, basic farmland transformation, control of soil erosion, agricultural power supply, drinking water for human and animals, local and remote relocation, agricultural product processing stations, agricultural service centers, agricultural vocational secondary schools, and so on. The proportion of poor households fell from 75 to 15%. The 10-year project explored an effective path and model for the development-oriented poverty alleviation in the poverty-stricken areas. In 1993, the central government decided to extend the project for another decade.

Source Gao (2014).

On May 16, 1986, the General Office of the State Council issued the *Notice on the Establishment of the State Council Leading Group of Economic Development in Poor Areas*, an inter-departmental coordinating and deliberative body under the State Council based on China's multidimensional definition of "poverty." The leading group office was set up to deal with specific affairs and was co-located with the "Three Western Areas Office." The leading group was composed of one leader—the Secretary-General of the State Council, three consultants, two deputy leaders—Vice

[2]The three western areas cover an area of 380,000 km^2, incorporating a total of 47 counties, including 19 in Hexi, 20 in Dingxi and 8 in Xihaigu, with an agricultural population of 12 million. With an annual precipitation less than 300 mm, these western areas suffer from drought and are among the most impoverished areas in China.

Chairman from the State Planning Commission and the State Science and Technology Commission, and members from 14 departments, including deputy heads of the State Education Commission, Ministry of Civil Affairs, Ministry of Finance, Ministry of Commerce, Ministry of Agriculture, Ministry of Forestry, Ministry of Water and Power, Ministry of Transport, Ministry of Health, Rural Development Research Center of the State Council, and Agricultural Bank of China, as well as the director of the Leading Group Office of Agricultural Development in Three Western Areas.[3]

Seen from the institutional setup of the leading group, it's under the leadership of the State Council, encompassing the State Planning Commission in charge of development planning, the Ministry of Finance for financial budget, the Agricultural Bank of China for discount loans, the ministries of agriculture, forestry, water, commerce and others to increase income of farmers, the Ministry of Transport for infrastructure, the ministries of education and health for key public services, the Ministry of Civil Affairs for disaster relief, the Rural Development Research Center of the State Council for policy research relating to agricultural development in China, as well as the Leading Group Office of Agricultural Development in Three Western Areas for policy research in agricultural development in western China. Such a cross-sector coordinating and deliberative institution gathered all the key departments for the fight against rural poverty. The establishment of dedicated institutions has contributed to the great progress in poverty reduction (see Box 4.2).

Box 4.2 Achievement of the first-stage development-oriented poverty reduction

Since the establishment of the State Council Leading Group of Economic Development in Poor Areas in 1986, the poor population (measured by the standard at the time) dropped from 125 million in 1985 to 80 million in 1992, registering an annual decrease of 6.4 million on average. As the poor population in the world remained at a high level through the 1980s, China's massive poverty reduction won wide acclaim from the international community. According to the World Bank's report "China: Strategies for Reducing Poverty in the 1990s" issued at the International Symposium on Poverty Alleviation in China held in October 1992, "The Chinese government has made great efforts to help the most backward rural areas get rid of poverty. These efforts have turned out to be much more successful than those in many other developing countries." Then Vice President Sven Sandstrom of the World Bank said at the symposium that the East Asia, with China playing a leading role, is the most successful in poverty reduction in the world. The proportion of the poor people in China fell from one-third to one-tenth, which has been unprecedented both in speed and in scale.

Source Zhang (2007a, b).

[3]General Office of the State Council (1986).

In 1993, the State Council decided to reorganize the State Council Leading Group of Economic Development in Poor Areas and renamed it the State Council Leading Group of Poverty Alleviation and Development. The new leading group was headed by a state councilor, with an enlarged team of deputy leaders from 20-plus institutions, featuring new ones like Research Office of the State Council, People's Bank of China, Ministry of Labor, Ministry of Foreign Trade, National Family Planning Commission, Central Committee of the Communist Youth League, All-China Federation of Trade Unions, All-China Women's Federation, China Association for Science and Technology and China Disabled Persons' Federation.[4] Compared with the leading group of economic development in poor areas that mainly involved government institutions in charge of infrastructure, agriculture, education and health, the new leading group attached importance to the foreign trade and employment, particularly the special institutions for women and children, the disabled and other special groups of poor people. It demonstrated an extended understanding of the connotations of poverty and led to expansion of relevant policies. Since then, the State Council Leading Group of Poverty Alleviation and Development has seen a growing body of member institutions with the expansion of the development-oriented poverty-reduction projects. In 2015, in an effort to win the battle against poverty by 2020, the Chinese government expanded the leading group to incorporate more than 40 government departments and organizations.

In addition to dedicated poverty-reduction institutions at the level of the central government, the provincial, municipal and county-level leading groups of development-oriented poverty reduction and corresponding offices were set up. In this way, a top-down and cross-sector poverty-reduction system was put in place. The central government is responsible for making overall plan, the provincial governments taking the overall responsibility and the cities and counties carrying it out. This specialized poverty-reduction agency across multiple government departments is dedicated to the development-oriented poverty alleviation targeting poor areas and poor people, as well as the correction of unfavorable conditions for poor areas and poor people in the market economy to deliver more benefits to the poor people.

4.3 Formulating Specific Strategies for Poverty Reduction

An important responsibility of the State Council Leading Group of Poverty Alleviation and Development is to study and formulate national strategies and policies for development-oriented poverty reduction. So far, China has implemented three specialized national poverty-reduction strategies.

[4]General Office of the State Council (1988).

4.3.1 The Seven-Year Program for Lifting 80 Million People Out of Poverty (1994–2000)

1. Background

China has since 1986 carried out planned, organized and large-scale development-oriented poverty reduction across the country. By the end of 1992, the number of rural poor had decreased from 250 million in 1978 to 80 million (in line with the 1978 rural poverty line). These poor people are mainly concentrated in 592 poverty-stricken counties targeted by the nation, distributed in the deep mountainous areas, rocky hills, desert areas, high-altitude and frigid areas, Loess Plateau, high-risk area of endemic diseases and reservoir areas, which are mostly former revolutionary base areas and ethnic minority regions. They all feature remoteness, inconvenient transportation, ecological imbalance, slow economic development, backward culture and education, difficult access to drinking water for people and animals, and extremely poor production and living conditions. This is the main battlefield for the fight against poverty.

2. Overall goal

In 1994, the Chinese government decided to implement the *Seven-Year Program for Lifting 80 Million People out of Poverty (1994–2000)*, in a bid to pool manpower as well as material and financial resources and mobilize all sectors of society for a massive fight against poverty. With a view to meeting the basic needs of 80 million poor people by the end of 2000, all-out efforts were made to strengthen the infrastructure construction in poverty-stricken areas and improve backward educational, cultural and health services. The Chinese government set a multidimensional poverty-reduction goal, with the focus on improving the production capacity and human capital from multiple aspects. It's the essence of development-oriented poverty alleviation. See Box 4.3 for details.

Box 4.3 Multidimensional poverty-reduction goals

Goal 1: Meet the basic needs of the poor people by the end of 2020.

Target 1.1: The annual per capita net income of most poverty-stricken households will reach RMB 500 (at 1990 constant prices).

Target 1.2: Help the poverty-stricken households to create the basic conditions to meet the basic needs in a sustainable way. Where possible, there should be 0.08–0.16 of per capita farmland with stably high yield, 0.16 of orchard or commercial crops for each household, one member from each household to be sent for work in firms in towns or other developed areas, one type of animal farming or domestic sideline occupation for each household, and a fenced pasture or "enclosed pasture" for each household in the pastoral area. At the same time, the existing achievement in poverty reduction must be maintained to prevent people from falling into poverty again.

Goal 2: Strengthen infrastructure development.

Target 2.1: Most of human and animals will have access to drinking water.

Target 2.2: Most poverty-stricken towns and townships will have access to local markets and the commodity producing areas will have access to highways.

Target 2.3: Provide electricity to all counties and most impoverished villages.

Goal 3: Improve the backward education, culture and health.

Target 3.1: Popularize primary education, and actively eliminate illiteracy among young people.

Target 3.2: Develop vocational and technical education and training for adults to make sure most young laborers master one or two practical skills.

Target 3.3: Improve medical and health conditions, prevent and treat endemic diseases, and prevent disability

Target 3.4: Strictly carry out family planning policy to bring the natural population growth rate within the limits set by the state

Source The Seven-Year Program for Lifting 80 Million People out of Poverty (1994–2000)

3. Guidelines

The government should follow the path of development-oriented poverty alleviation, encourage the officials and residents in poverty-stricken areas to take initiative and work hard to meet their subsistence needs and eventually get rid of poverty by developing local resources and commodities with the help of government support and technologies, in a market-oriented way.

4. Methods

To begin with, develop agricultural industry, with the focus on plant and animal farming and related processing, transportation and marketing industries featuring low investment, quick returns and high yields that are conducive to meet the basic needs of the poor directly. Second, develop village and township enterprises based on resources endowment and competitive edge. Efforts should be made to develop resource-developing and labor-intensive enterprises that could give full play to the resource advantages of the impoverished areas and provide job opportunities for the poor people. Third, reform the land system. By means of land lease and transfer of rights to use the land, accelerate the exploitation and utilization of the wasteland, barren hills, slopes and beaches, as well as wastewater. Fourth, transfer rural work-force. Planned and organized export of labor services shall be conducted to transfer the labor forces in poverty-stricken areas in a rational and orderly manner. Fifth, alleviate poverty through relocation. The development-oriented relocation shall be carried out for villages and rural households suffering from harsh conditions for survival and development.

5. Funds

There are three types of poverty-reduction funds: government funds, credit funds and work relief funds. The government funds for poverty reduction are mainly used for projects with better social benefits; credit funds for development projects with better economic returns and capacity for repayment of loans; and the work relief funds for roads, water conservancy projects and providing safe drinking water for people and animals.

6. Policy guarantee

The policies fall into three categories. The first category refers to the policies for concessional loans. Under the premise of guaranteed economic benefits and repayment capacity, the poor households and economic entities engaged in poverty reduction enjoy appropriately broadened access to credit funds. State-owned commercial banks must earmark a certain amount of credit funds each year to selectively support some projects with good economic returns and repayment capacity in poverty-stricken areas. The second category refers to the policies for fiscal and tax incentives. The newly established firms in the "former revolutionary bases, ethnic minority enclaves, border and impoverished" areas designated by the state could have the income tax fully or partially refunded within three years. Governments at all levels have included poverty-reduction funds in their budgets to ensure their use for development-oriented poverty reduction. Appropriate subsidies are given to poor households who lived on resold grain. The third category refers to the preferential policies for economic development. While planning development projects, the central and local governments should give priority to poor areas with better resource conditions, and while formulating and implementing industrial policies, to the poor areas. When it comes to the imports and exports, when other conditions are the same, priority support should be given to poverty-stricken areas.

7. Department-specific tasks

The Seven-Year Program for Lifting 80 Million People out of Poverty (1994–2000) assigned poverty-reduction tasks for dozens of departments in planning, domestic and foreign trade, agriculture, forestry, water, science and education, transportation, railway, electric power, mining, coal, metallurgy, building materials, chemicals, post and telecommunications, labor, civil affairs, ethnic minorities, culture, health, family planning, finance, industry and commerce, customs and others. After dividing these departments into different groups, the author found that the program mainly aims to support the development of rural infrastructure, key public services for the formation of human capital, agricultural production, processing and trade, and transfer of employment of labor forces.

8. Social mobilization

Following the launch of *the Seven-Year Program for Lifting 80 Million People out of Poverty (1994–2000)*, China has initially set up a mechanism to mobilize all sectors of the society for development-oriented poverty reduction. First, the eastern developed regions are asked to help the poor areas in the west. The developed regions are mobilized to provide financial assistance to the impoverished areas in the west. Boasting advantages in technology, talent, market, information and material resources, the companies in the developed regions are encouraged to cooperate with those in the west for mutual benefits in the forms of economic cooperation, technological service, labor employment and product proliferation, just to name a few. In addition, official and talent exchanges between the east and the west are encouraged. Second, the central and local Party and government offices as well as qualified enterprises and public institutions are required to link them with certain poverty-stricken counties for poverty reduction. Third, junior colleges, universities and research institutes are required to fully leverage their advantages in talent and technology for poverty reduction in poor areas. Fourth, the other political parties, All-China Federation of Industry and Commerce, the trade unions, the Communist Youth League, women's federations, disabled persons' federations, China Foundation for Poverty Alleviation and other civil organizations are all mobilized for poverty alleviation.

The *Seven-Year Program for Lifting 80 Million People out of Poverty (1994–2000)* is the first program of action for development-oriented poverty reduction with clarified objectives, targets, measures and deadlines. It put in place the institutional framework and foundation for China's development-oriented poverty alleviation. Start from improving infrastructure and public services in poverty-stricken areas before increasing agricultural productivity and transferring employment of labor forces in these areas. Development-oriented poverty alleviation targeting poor areas and people aims to ease poverty and improve the living standards of poor people from multiple perspectives. In addition, the institutional frameworks for the east–west collaboration in poverty alleviation as well as the targeted poverty alleviation for government departments, enterprises and public institutions were established. The mechanism for mobilization of all sectors of society, including social organizations, has taken shape. Throughout the process of development-oriented poverty alleviation, the government has played a leading role in the formulation of strategies, plans and policies and has developed a powerful poverty-governance model based on cross-sector coordination. See Box 4.4 for the achievements of the *Seven-Year Program for Lifting 80 Million People out of Poverty (1994–2000).*

Box 4.4 Achievements of the *Seven-Year Program for Lifting 80 Million People out of Poverty (1994–2000)*

The *Seven-Year Program for Lifting 80 Million People out of Poverty (1994–2000)* has achieved the following results. First, the poor population decreased rapidly. Measured against China's rural poverty line at the time, the poor population dropped from 80 million in 1992 to 32.09 million in 2000, while the incidence of poverty fell from 8.8 to 3.5%. Second, the infrastructure in poor villages improved significantly. By the end of 2000, the proportion of administrative villages with access to electricity, roads, postal services and landlines reached 95.5, 89, 69 and 67.7%, respectively. Third, the poverty-stricken counties experienced rapid economic growth. During the program period, the agricultural added value of the national poverty-stricken counties increased by 54%, with an average annual growth rate of 7.5%; the industrial added value increased by 99.3%, with an average annual growth of 12.2%; the local fiscal revenue nearly doubled, with an average annual growth of 12.9%; the grain output increased by 12.3%, with an average annual growth of 1.9%; and per capita net income of farmers increased from RMB 648 to RMB 1,337, with an average annual growth of 12.8%. Fourth, the population and human capital in poverty-stricken areas increased markedly. The momentum of excessive population growth in poverty-stricken areas was curbed, evidenced by a declining natural population growth rate. The school conditions were improved. Among a total of 592 key counties for poverty alleviation, 318 counties provided nine-year compulsory education and basically eliminated illiteracy among young people. Vocational and adult education developed rapidly, which improved the quality of labor forces effectively. In most poor areas, township hospitals were renovated or rebuilt and poor medical services improved. A large number of practical agricultural technologies were promoted to help farmers farm in a more scientific way.

4.3.2 *The* Outline for Development-Oriented Poverty Alleviation for China's Rural Areas (2001–2010)

Following the notable success of the *Seven-Year Program for Lifting 80 Million People out of Poverty (1994–2000)*, the Chinese government decided to formulate a new decade-long national poverty-reduction strategy and came up with the *Outline for Development-Oriented Poverty Alleviation for China's Rural Areas (2001–2010)*.

1. Overall goal

The overall goal is to meet the basic needs of a small number of poor people as soon as possible, further improve the basic production and living conditions in poverty-stricken areas, consolidate the results gained in this regard, improve the poor people's quality of life and comprehensive quality, speed up the construction of infrastructure facilities in impoverished rural areas, improve the ecological environment and gradually overcome the economic, social and cultural backwardness in the poverty-stricken areas, and create conditions for building a moderately prosperous society.

2. Guidelines

First, poverty alleviation should be done in a development-oriented way. With the focus on economic development, the people in the poverty-stricken areas are guided to leverage the national assistance and support, respond to market demand, adjust economic structure, explore local resources, develop commodity production and improve production conditions. As productivity increases, the poor households will have greater capacities for self-accumulation and self-development. Second, pursue the policy of integrated and all-round development. By incorporating development-oriented poverty reduction into the national economic and social development plans, the government shall strengthen infrastructure construction, such as water conservancy, transportation, electric power, communications; attach importance to the development of science and technology, education, health and culture; improve the community environment and the quality of life; and promote coordinated socioeconomic development and progress in all respects in poverty-stricken areas. Third, development should be sustainable. Poverty alleviation and development must be combined with resource and ecological conservation and family planning, to control the excessive growth of population in poverty-stricken areas, achieve a virtuous cycle between resources, population and environment, and improve the ability for sustainable development in poverty-stricken areas. Fourth, self-reliance and hard work should be encouraged as always. The government should give full play to the enthusiasm and creativity of the officials and people in poverty-stricken areas, strive for self-improvement with perseverance, and rely on their own strength to overcome the backwardness and poverty. Fifth, government leadership and social participation should be adhered to. The government should actively mobilize and organize all sectors of society to support the development and construction of poverty-stricken areas by multiple means.

3. Targets and priorities

First, targets. Poverty alleviation and development targets the poor population in poverty-stricken areas struggling to meet their basic needs for survival, as well as the poor people who have met their basic needs so as to help them increase income, improve production and living conditions, and consolidate the results in this regard. Second, priorities. Having contiguous impoverished areas in the sight, the Chinese government made the ethnic minority regions in central and western China, former revolutionary base areas, border areas and impoverished areas the priorities for development-oriented poverty reduction and identified key counties in these four types of areas for development-oriented poverty reduction. Third, poverty-reduction plans. With the county as the basic unit, the plans clearly defined the goals, contents, measures, support units and funding sources for the development-oriented poverty reduction of the poor villages.

4. Methods

First, develop plant and animal farming as a key method for development-oriented poverty reduction. Strengths should be gathered to help the poor people to develop distinctive plant and animal farming to meet the market demands and increase their income. It should be oriented toward sustainable development based on the ecological conservation and improvement. Second, actively promote agricultural industrialization. In the direction of industrialized development, contiguous impoverished area should be viewed as a whole for the planning to develop dominant industry with local features. Efforts should be made to actively develop "company + farmer" model and contract farming. Large and medium-sized agricultural product processing companies should be directed and encouraged to establish raw material production bases in poverty-stricken areas, provide pre-, mid- and post-production services for poor rural households and develop industrialized operation featuring integration of trade, industry and agriculture as well as that of production, supply and marketing. Efforts should be reinforced in the construction of agricultural product wholesale markets in poverty-stricken areas, to further invigorate circulation, and gradually form a large-scale and specialized production pattern. Third, improve the basic production and living conditions in poor areas. The construction of basic farmland, infrastructure, environmental renovation and public service facilities should be strengthened in poverty-stricken townships and villages. Fourth, increase efforts to alleviate poverty through science and technology. The government should take full advantage of technological resources and advancements, stimulate the enthusiasm of scientists and engineers, encourage them to start businesses in poverty-stricken areas and accelerate the technological application. It should also establish demonstration bases for poverty reduction through science and technology, and focus on the demonstration effect and give full play to the leading role of science and technology in development-oriented poverty reduction. Fifth, strive to improve the scientific and technological literacy of the people in poverty-stricken areas. The government should make all-out efforts to enhance basic education and raise the education level of the poor in general; provide targeted vocational and technical education and short-term training to help farmers' master advanced and practical technology. Sixth, actively and steadily expand the export of labor services from poverty-stricken areas. The government should strengthen the vocational skills training of the labor force in these areas, while organizing and directing the migration of labor forces in a healthy and orderly manner. Developed coastal areas, as well as large and medium-sized cities, should give priority to workers from impoverished areas, when other conditions are the same. Seventh, make steady efforts in voluntary relocation of the poor people. Efforts should be made to move them to and settle them in new homes and increase their income. Eighth, encourage the economic entities of diverse ownerships to participate in development-oriented poverty reduction.

Since the release of the new 10-year outline for development-oriented poverty alleviation, the Chinese government has stepped up efforts in development-oriented poverty alleviation and elevated it as a part of national strategy toward building a moderately prosperous society in all respects and achieving common prosperity for everyone. See Box 4.5 for China's achievements in poverty reduction (2001–2010).

Box 4.5 China's achievements in poverty reduction (2001–2010)

Thanks to the implementation of the new decade-long outline for poverty reduction, China made continuous achievements in multidimensional poverty reduction. First, the poor population decreased dramatically. In line with the rural poverty line in 2010 at RMB 1,274 for per capita net income of farmers on a yearly basis, the number of rural poor in China fell from 94.22 million at the end of 2000 to 26.88 million at the end of 2010. The proportion of rural poor to the total rural population dropped from 10.2% in 2000 to 2.8% in 2010. Second, the industrial structure in poor areas was further optimized; specialty and competitive industries developed rapidly; and the comprehensive economic strength of poor counties grew constantly. From 2001 to 2010, 592 key counties in the national development-oriented poverty–reduction programs saw their per capita gross regional product grow from RMB 2,658 to RMB 11,170, registering an average annual growth of 17%. The per capita net income of farmers grew from RMB 1,276 in 2001 to RMB 3,273 in 2010, with an average annual increase of 11% (not factoring in the inflation). All these figures are all higher than the national average. Third, production and living conditions in poor areas were greatly improved. From 2002 to 2010, 592 key counties in the national development-oriented poverty-reduction programs saw their basic farmland increase by 52.456 million, and the mileage of newly constructed, renovated and extended roads by 952,000 km. By the end of 2010, in the key counties in the national development-oriented poverty-reduction programs, 60.9% of rural households had access to tap water or well water, 88.1% of villages had access to roads, 98% had access to electricity and 92.9% had access to landlines. In addition, their per capita housing space reached 24.9 m^2, and 88.4% of the rural households had sanitary latrines or flush toilets. Fourth, social undertakings in poor areas made constant progress. By the end of 2010, in the key counties, 97.7% of children aged between 7 and 15 were enrolled in school, close to the national average level; the illiteracy rate of young and middle-aged people had decreased to 7, 5.4% points lower than in 2002; and the average schooling time for the young and middle-aged had reached eight years. By the end of 2010, in the key counties, 93.3% of rural households were covered by the new cooperative medical care system, and 91.4% of rural residents had access to timely medical service; every township had a hospital, and most administrative villages had a clinic. Fifth, ecological degradation was brought under initial control. From 2002 to 2010, in the key counties, 149.235 million of low-yield farmland was restored to forest or grassland, and a total of 226.434 million of land was newly covered by commercial forest. In these counties, the proportion of households whose drinking water sources were polluted decreased from

15.5% in 2002 to 5.1% in 2010, and that of households having difficult access to fuel decreased from 45 to 31.4%.

Source Information Office of the State Council (2011).

4.3.3 The Outline for Development-Oriented Poverty Reduction for China's Rural Areas (2011–2020)

1. Overall goal

By 2020, the state is committed to ensuring that the impoverished rural population has stable access to adequate food and clothing, compulsory education, and basic medical services and housing; to realizing a growth rate of per capita net income in poor rural areas higher than the national average; to achieving indices of major basic public services close to the national average levels; and to putting a brake on the widening development gap.

The overall goal could be interpreted from the following aspects. First, it's a multidimensional poverty-reduction goal. The "stable access to adequate food and clothing" addresses the basic needs of the poor people, while "compulsory education, basic medical services and housing" are associated with the basic capabilities of the poor people. Education and health put more emphasis on long-term investment in human capital. Second, it aims at pro-poor growth by "realizing a growth rate of per-capita net income in poor rural areas higher than the national average." Third, it's oriented toward inclusive development by "achieving indices of major basic public services close to the national average levels and putting a brake on the widening development gap." The overall goal demonstrated China's further progress in the concept of development-oriented poverty alleviation.

2. Main tasks

The *Outline for Development-oriented Poverty Reduction for China's Rural Areas (2011–2020)* sets 12 main tasks in four categories. The first category relates to infrastructure, covering five tasks in basic farmland and irrigation, safe drinking water, electric power for household and production purposes, transportation and renovation of dilapidated housing in rural areas. The second category is about public services, incorporating five tasks concerning education, medical services, public culture, social security, as well as population and family planning. The third category is linked with industrial development—the task of developing specialty and competitive industries. The fourth is for ecological conservation, planned to increase the forest coverage by 3.5% points by 2020 compared with that at the end of 2010.

3. Targets

The outline targets at poor population, poor villages, 592 impoverished counties and 14 contiguous impoverished areas.

4. Three-Pronged Poverty Alleviation Scheme

The *Outline for Poverty Reduction and Development for China's Rural Areas (2011–2020)* put forward a three-pronged poverty alleviation scheme that consists of special action plans, sectoral programs and society-wide poverty-reduction initiatives. Special action plans for poverty-stricken areas and populations aim at specific poverty-reduction goals, such as relocating the poor people who lived in inhospitable areas, comprehensive development-oriented poverty reduction in villages, work in lieu of aids, promoting the agrobusiness development, boosting employment, implementing pilot projects and promoting the development of former revolutionary bases. Sectoral programs are projects designed and executed orchestrated by government bodies and industrial sectors, including development of local niche industries, poverty reduction through science and technology, infrastructure improvement, development of education and culture, improvement of public health and population management, improvement of the social security system, and energy and ecology projects. Society-wide poverty-reduction initiatives work by establishing one-to-one partnerships aimed at facilitating the movement of development aid, economic cooperation and personnel exchange between the Central Party Committee and state organs, SOEs and public institutions in economically developed areas in eastern China and beneficiaries in poverty-stricken areas in western China. Contributions by the military and armed forces, and voluntary services of enterprises and social organizations would also fall under this category. The different components of the poverty alleviation and development scheme are shown in Fig. 4.2.

5. Policy guarantee

The *Outline for Development-oriented Poverty Reduction for China's Rural Areas (2011–2020)* further specified the special national policies targeting the poverty-stricken areas and poor population in terms of investment, finance and tax, financial services, industrial support, land use and ecological conservation. It strongly emphasized to include development-oriented poverty-reduction schemes for ethnic minorities, women, children and the disabled in its planning, make unified arrangements for their implementation, give priority to their implementation when all conditions are equal and strengthen support for these groups. See Box 4.6 for the outcomes of the Outline.

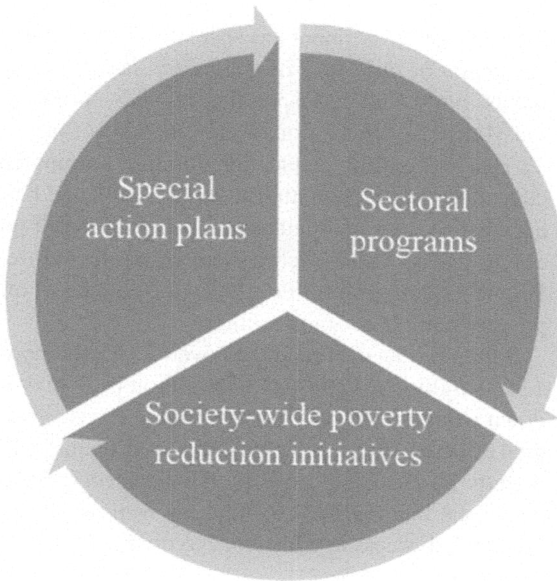

Fig. 4.2 China's poverty reduction and development scheme

Box 4.6 Outcomes of the *Outline for Development-oriented Poverty Reduction for China's Rural Areas (2011–2020)*

Following the launch of the *Outline for Development-oriented Poverty Reduction for China's Rural Areas (2011–2020)*, the Chinese government has made a raft of new measures in this regard. To begin with, it adjusted the rural poverty line to an annual income of RMB 2,300 at the constant price in 2000, equivalent to USD 2.29 per person per day (2011 PPP). Second, plans for regional development and poverty reduction were formulated respectively for 14 contiguous impoverished areas. Third, it's proposed to "continue the war against poverty" and lift all people living below the current poverty line out of poverty. Further, the Chinese government has put forward the strategy of targeted poverty reduction and eradication. With the household as the basic unit, the government proposed to identify poor households of the remaining 89 million poor people one by one, create separate files, analyze the reasons for their poverty, find out their needs, formulate plans and take targeted measures to shake off poverty on a case-by-case basis. Fifth, the Chinese government commissioned a third-party agency in 2016 to conduct independent evaluation of the accuracy in identifying the poor households and in poverty delisting, people's satisfaction with the poverty reduction work, based on a stratified random sampling of 1‰ from 22 provinces with poor population, measured as people living below the national poverty line. Sixth, the Chinese government assessed the performance of provincial Party committees and governments in poverty reduction and developed corresponding measures. Seventh, the Chinese government has specially drawn up the *National Plan for Poverty Reduction in the 13th Five-Year Plan Period*. Eighth, all government departments introduced corresponding policies on poverty reduction. For example, the Ministry of Education offered the kids of registered poor households with 12-year compulsory education for free (compared with 9-year compulsory education nationwide); the National Health and Family Planning Commission established a special database for the registered poverty-stricken households due to diseases and offered them with targeted treatment and assistance; the People's Bank of China developed the policies of microloans and relending for poverty reduction, among others.

Measured against the new poverty line, the poor population dropped from 122.38 million in 2011 to 55.75 million in 2015, with the incidence of poverty down from 12.7 to 5.7%. The Chinese government set the poverty-reduction goal of lifting all poor people, measured against the current poverty line, out of poverty by 2020. The poverty delisting criteria involve an income sustainably above the national poverty line, as well as adequate food and clothing and guaranteed access to education, basic medical service and housing.

4.4 Promoting Region-Wide Development-Oriented Poverty Reduction

Targeting poverty-stricken areas to reduce poverty on a large scale through regional development has always been an important part of development-oriented poverty reduction with Chinese characteristics. In 1986, there were 331 nationally designated poor counties and 333 provincially or regionally designated poor counties, among which 64.8% were concentrated in 18 contiguous impoverished areas across the country. In 2001, the State Council Leading Group Office of Poverty Alleviation and Development compiled *A Chronicle of Development-oriented Poverty Reduction in Rural China (1978–2000)*. Therefore, targeting the poverty-stricken counties to fight against poverty on a large scale through regional development has long been a main strategy for China's development-oriented poverty reduction.

The *Outline for Development-oriented Poverty Reduction for China's Rural Areas (2011–2020)* specified 14 contiguous impoverished areas as the main battlefield for development-oriented poverty reduction in the new decade. The Plan for Regional Development and Poverty Reduction in Contiguous Impoverished Areas was drawn up accordingly. Such strategy is based on the fact that the regional poverty in China presents some obvious common features. Despite various priorities for development of different regions associated with natural conditions, geological locations and socioeconomic development levels, the development of these contiguous areas shares the following features.

4.4.1 *Infrastructure Connectivity*

On July 13, 2013, the Ministry of Transport issued the *Outline on Poverty Reduction through Transportation Construction in Contiguous Impoverished Areas (2011–2020)*. The construction of transportation infrastructure covers expressways, national and provincial trunk lines, as well as rural roads. First, the expressway construction shall focus on national expressways to connect the broken roads and bottleneck sections of the important passages. During the 12th Five-Year Plan period, roughly 10,700 km of expressway shall be built. Second, in terms of the national and provincial trunk lines, Grade II highways shall be built into counties to enhance connections within the region and with the outside world. During the 12th Five-Year Plan period, roughly 29,000 km of such trunk lines shall be built. Third, regarding rural roads, tarmac and cement roads shall be built in administrative villages, along with necessary safety and protection facilities and medium and small-span bridges. During the same period, about 10,700 and 222,000 km of tarmac and cement roads shall be built in a total of 419 townships and 39,164 administrative villages, respectively. Approximately 17,000 km of roads in counties to develop tourism and resource exploitation shall be built, with a view to facilitating the socioeconomic development in the poor areas.

The *13th Five-Year Plan for Poverty Reduction through Transportation Construction* further specified that by 2020, a network of national trunk expressways shall be basically put in place. Where conditions permit, county seats shall have access to highways of Grade II and above, and townships and administrative villages have tarmac or cement roads and complete access to bus services. These efforts aim to build a safe and convenient transport system with well-connected roads extending to townships and villages and bus services covering villages, laying a solid foundation for the building of a moderately prosperous society in all respects and leaving no place behind due to lack in the access to transportation facilities.

4.4.2 *Equitable Access to Public Services*

The main goal concerning equitable access to public services is to achieve, by 2020, indices of major basic public services close to the national average levels.[5] To this end, a series of policies in education, health and other basic public services have been introduced.

1. Education policies

First, the Ministry of Education introduced the policy of providing living subsidies to teachers working in contiguous impoverished rural areas. By the end of 2015,

[5]The Decision of the CPC Central Committee and the State Council on Eradicating Poverty in China (Zhong Fa (2015).

the policy had been implemented in 573 counties or 82% of counties in contiguous impoverished areas, benefiting 71,000 schools and 10.44 million teachers working in rural areas, with a coverage rate of 96 and 92%, respectively.[6] Second, the Nutrition Improvement Plan for Rural Students Receiving Compulsory Education has been initiated since the fall semester of 2011, beginning with pilot projects in contiguous areas in dire needs. The central government launched a program of nutrition improvement for rural students receiving compulsory education, offering a nutritious meal allowance of RMB 3 per day per student in impoverished areas, with the pilot project covering about 26 million students in 680 counties. Today, the allowance has been raised to RMB 4 per day per student, covering all contiguous impoverished areas. Third, the Ministry of Education, the National Development and Reform Commission and the Ministry of Finance jointly issued the *Opinions on Overall Improvement of the Conditions of Disadvantaged Schools of Compulsory Education in Poverty-stricken Areas* for an all-round renovation of the school buildings and facilities.

2. Health policies

First, in 2012, the Ministry of Health and the All-China Women's Federation (ACWF) jointly carried out the pilot nutrition improvement program for children in poor areas. With the specialized subsidies allocated by the central government, free nutrition packages were provided to infants aged 6–24 months, with a view to prevent malnutrition and anemia in infants and promote healthy growth of infants in poverty-stricken areas.[7] Second, in 2016, the National Health and Family Planning Commission, the State Council Leading Group of Poverty Alleviation and Development and 13 other departments jointly launched *Guiding Opinions on Implementing Poverty Reduction through Health Promotion* and initiated a series of policies in this regard.[8] See Chap. 5 for elaboration of these details.[9] Third, special polices were introduced for capacity building to prevent and control diseases in Tibet.

4.4.3 Poverty Reduction Through Ecological Conservation

In response to the environmental problems facing China as well as the UN's 2030 Sustainable Development Goals, the CPC Central Committee put forward the concept of "green development" and dedicated a chapter to "poverty eradication through

[6]Circular of the General Office of the Ministry of Education on the Implementation of Living Subsidies for Teachers Working in Contiguous Impoverished Rural Areas. Teachers' Affairs Department [2016] No.4. March 11, 2016.

[7]Notice of the Ministry of Health on Promulgation of the Management Plan for the Pilot Nutrition Improvement Program for Children in Poor Areas. By Ministry of Health and ACWF [2012] No.276. 2012.

[8]Guiding Opinions on Implementing Poverty Alleviation through Health Promotion. By Financial Department of the National Health and Family Planning Commission. [2016] No.26. June 2016.

[9]Policies on poverty alleviation through health promotion are elaborated in Chap. 5.

ecological conservation" in the *National Plan for Poverty Reduction in the 13th Five-Year Plan Period*. The goal is to properly handle the relationship between ecological conservation and development-oriented poverty reduction, strengthen ecological conservation and rehabilitation in poverty-stricken areas, and improve their sustainable development capacity. Continuous efforts shall be made to expand the ecological compensation in poor areas, create more ecological conservation jobs, and with them help the poor people get rid of poverty.[10]

1. Implement major ecological conservation projects to alleviate poverty and strengthen ecological restoration

Major ecological conservation projects in China include the Grain for Green Program, pastureland-to-grassland project, the second-phase ecological conservation and construction project at the headwaters of the Yangtze, Yellow and Lancang rivers in Qinghai Province, Beijing and Tianjin sandstorm source control project, the project of forest shelterbelts in northwest-north-northeast China, the protection project of natural forest resources, key projects for soil and water conservation, the project to reverse the trend of desertification in Karst areas, the project of enclosed reserves of desertified land, the wetland protection and restoration project, as well as comprehensive management of grassland reclamation in the transition zone between cropping area and nomadic area. These projects mainly address regional ecological problems and focus on special treatment in combination with development-oriented poverty reduction. It's a national plan that integrates poverty reduction with sustainable development, the fastest and largest-scale action toward the fulfillment of the UN's 2030 sustainable development goals, as well as the first national plan that associate poverty eradication with sustainable development. See Box 4.7 for details about the Grain for Green Program.

Box 4.7 Grain for Green Program

Widespread deforestation and crop growing on hillsides and sandy land resulted in serious soil erosion and frequent natural disasters such as flood, draught and sandstorm, producing a serious impact on the productive activities and life of the people, and threatening the ecological security of the country. In response, China initiated on a trial basis the Grain for Green Program in Sichuan, Shaanxi and Gansu provinces in 1999, and expanded it to more areas in 2000. The program was carried out in a total of 1,897 counties in 25 provinces (municipalities, autonomous regions) between 2001 and 2010, and converted 28,577,200 hectares of farmland to forest from 1999 to 2014. Based on the estimate in 2014, it generated ecological benefits that were worth RMB 1.0072 trillion in 13 provinces in the upper and middle reaches of Yangtze River and the Yellow River. In the areas where the program was implemented, the financial subsidy

---

[10]Notice of the State Council on Promulgation of the National Plan for Poverty Alleviation in the 13th Five-Year Plan Period (2016).

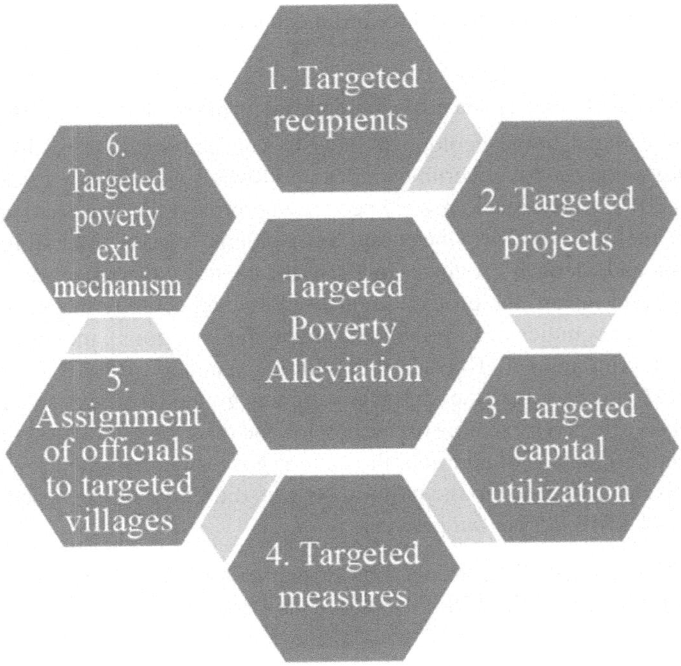
1. Targeted recipients
2. Targeted projects
3. Targeted capital utilization
4. Targeted measures
5. Assignment of officials to targeted villages
6. Targeted poverty exit mechanism
Targeted Poverty Alleviation

Fig. 4.3 Implications of targeted poverty reduction

in China; we need a more effective mechanism targeting poor households and poor people. In this context, the CPC Central Committee and the State Council came up with the strategy of targeted poverty reduction.

4.5.1 Implications

The implications of targeted poverty reduction can be interpreted from six aspects, as shown in Fig. 4.3. First, targeted measures in terms of recipients. Based on the poverty identification with the basic unit of household beginning in 2014, some 29 million households and over 88 million people were identified as poverty-stricken.[12] The statistics have been updated on a yearly basis. These identified poor households were registered in file, incorporating information about the family members, production and living conditions, income, reasons for poverty, needs to get rid of poverty, among others. Second, targeted measures in terms of projects. Relevant local government departments were required to match poverty-reduction projects with poor households and poor people. Third, targeted measures in terms of funding.

[12]Notable Progress in China's Development-oriented Poverty Alleviation in 2014: Targeted Measures for Root Cause of Poverty. *Guangming Daily*. January 30, 2015.

The poverty-reduction fund should be used for poor households and poor people to maximize the benefits and yields of the fund. Fourth, every impoverished household is guaranteed help. The measures should help address the reasons for poverty of each household and meet their respective needs to get rid of poverty. Fifth, every village has designated officials to carry out poverty eradication measures. One Party secretary and two or three officials shall be sent to each of the 128,000 identified poor villages for special poverty-reduction programs. These officials were generally selected from government departments, SOEs and public institutions in townships, counties, cities and provinces, as well as the banking system, similar to social workers. Sixth, poverty-reduction goals are met within the defined standards. Inspection and verification shall be carried out for each household that got rid of poverty for a guarantee of the effect.

4.5.2 Goals

By 2020, the state is committed to ensuring that the impoverished rural population has stable access to adequate food and clothing, compulsory education, and basic medical services and housing; to realizing a growth rate of per capita disposable income in poor rural areas higher than the national average; to achieving indices of major basic public services close to the national average levels; to ensuring that the rural population living below the current poverty threshold and all impoverished counties are all lifted out of poverty; and to solving the problems of regional poverty.[13]

From the perspective of development, China's poverty-reduction goal by 2020 can be interpreted from following aspects. First, deliver more benefits to the poor population through pro-poor growth. Second, through equitable access to compulsory education, basic medical care services and other public services, promote inclusive development and lay a solid foundation for the poor population to shake off long-term poverty and prevent the intergenerational transmission of poverty. Third, reduce multidimensional poverty—income-based and non-income-based (compulsory education, basic medical care and housing) poverty—and overcome obstacles for building a moderately prosperous society in all aspects (see Fig. 4.4).

4.5.3 Fundamental Principles

In 2013, General-Secretary Jinping Xi of the CPC Central Committee proposed to implement the strategy of targeted poverty reduction based on the following six fundamental principles, giving prominence to the idea of development-oriented poverty reduction befitting the new circumstances.

---

[13]The Decision of the CPC Central Committee and the State Council on Eradicating Poverty in China (Zhong Fa (2015) No.34) (2015).

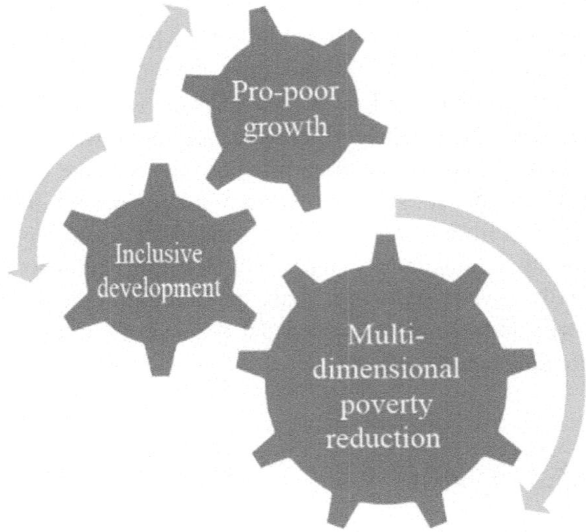

Fig. 4.4 China's poverty elimination goal by 2020

1. Uphold the Party leadership and consolidate the organizational foundation. Party chiefs at five levels of the state, province, municipality, county and village shall work together to reduce poverty.
2. Uphold the government guidance and enhance social cohesion. The government responsibilities should be strengthened to better guide all sectors of the society to make concerted efforts, and mobilize the rich to help the poor, so as to put in place an overall poverty-reduction system integrating special poverty-reduction programs, poverty reduction through industrial development and social involvement in poverty reduction.
3. Pursue the strategy of targeted poverty reduction and improve the effects in this regard. The government should properly address the problems concerning the recipients, implementers and methods of poverty reduction, in a bid to help the poor in need, achieve actual progress in poverty reduction, lift the poor out of poverty, make sustainable achievement in poverty reduction and deliver more benefits to the poor population.
4. Take the path of ecological conservation and green development. We must realize that lucid waters and lush mountains are invaluable assets and give priority to ecological conservation. The development-oriented poverty reduction shall not be carried out at the cost of the ecology. We shall explore a new path of poverty reduction through ecological conservation and restoration while helping the poor benefit more from this.
5. Give full play to the key role of the people and stimulate their internal impetus. We shall continue to promote development-oriented poverty reduction, properly handle the relationship between national support, social assistance and individual effort, carry forward the spirit of self-reliance, hard work and diligence, fully

mobilize the enthusiasm and creativity of the officials and people in poverty-stricken areas, enhance the skills of the impoverished population, and improve their capacity for self-development.

6. Tailor policies to local conditions and innovate systems and mechanisms. We should seek innovations in the problem-oriented methods for poverty reduction; make innovative use of poverty reduction resources, with a shift from distributed to intensive trend; innovate the model of development-oriented poverty reduction, with the focus shifting from "providing assistance" to "helping them to develop on their own"; innovate the poverty-reduction evaluation system, with the focus shifting from local output value to the achievements in poverty reduction.

4.5.4 Targeted Poverty-Reduction Programs

With a view to effectively carrying out targeted poverty reduction, the CPC Central Committee and the State Council came up with a range of poverty-reduction programs reflecting the characteristics of the poor population, the reasons of poverty and their needs to get rid of poverty. These programs could be broadly divided into four categories: programs to increase income and employment, public service programs, infrastructure programs and ecological conservation programs.

1. Special poverty-reduction programs to increase income and employment

First, develop industries with local features. We will focus on supporting poor villages and households to develop plant and animal farming and traditional handicraft industries based on local resource endowments and advantages. We will support the poverty-stricken areas to develop agricultural products processing industry, and accelerate the integrated development of the primary, secondary and tertiary industries, while delivering more value-added income from entire agricultural industry chain and value chain to the poor households. Second, guide the export of rural labor services. We'll invest more in labor training oriented toward employment to provide more targeted and effective training. We'll step up efforts in vocational skills training and poor households training to make sure that the poor family members master at least one skill to make a living. Efforts shall be made to strengthen the contact between the exporter and importer of rural migrant workers; foster the development of industries like home services, logistics and elderly care; expand job opportunities for the transfer of rural labor force; and enhance the policy support for the migrant workers to return hometown and start business. Third, carry out experiments on poverty reduction through asset investments. With poverty reduction as the ultimate goal, poverty-reduction funds and other funds for rural areas are invested in agriculture, aquaculture, photovoltaic, hydropower and rural tourism, and the resulting assets are quantified as shares owned by the poor villages and poor households, especially the ones with inability to work. We shall encourage the farmers' cooperatives and other business entities to help poor households to increase income, by placing their land and livestock under trusteeship and allowing them to make investment with their land management rights; support the development of hydropower, mineral resources and other resources in poverty-stricken areas and provide collective equity to villages whose land was occupied, so that the poor people can share the benefits of resource development.

2. Public service programs for poverty reduction

First, focus on poverty reduction through education. The government shall allocate more national education funds to poor areas and basic education; provide assistance to poor rural families so that their children could receive preschool education; steadily promote the nutrition improvement plan for poor rural students in compulsory education; step up effort to improve the qualification of rural teachers, offer cost-of-living subsidies to rural teachers in contiguous impoverished areas, and set up a system of honors for rural teachers. It should also improve the retention rate of compulsory education, and popularize senior-high-school education. Students from registered families with financial difficulties shall be exempt from tuition and other fees during senior high schools and secondary vocational schools. Secondary vocational education should be offered to the junior high school graduates who failed to get to senior high schools. Subsidies should be increased for college students from poor families and help offered for college graduates from poor families to find a job. Second, provide medical services and assistance to reduce poverty. Related programs are carried out to ensure basic medical and health services for the poor population so that they are not reduced to or returned to poverty because of illness. Financial subsidies are provided to reimburse the payment of the poor people covered by the New Rural Cooperative Medical System (NRCMS). The government should provide medical relief to all the poor people suffering from severe or major illnesses, guaranteeing medical treatment of major diseases for the poor; establish health files for the poor; provide medical treatment by category and implement treatment-before-payment policies for the poor people suffering from major diseases; take targeted measures to strengthen prevention and treatment of infectious diseases, endemic diseases and chronic diseases in poverty-stricken areas; implement across the board the nutrition improvement programs for the poor rural children, free neonatal screening, free cervical and breast cancer screenings for women, free prepregnancy health checkups, and other major public health programs. Third, implement and improve the system of subsistence allowance in rural areas. The households that cannot get rid of poverty through industrial or employment support shall be lifted out of poverty through subsistence allowances. The rural areas with lower standard of subsistence allowances shall gradually catch up with the national standard. Plan should be developed for effective integration of rural subsistence allowance system with development-oriented poverty-reduction policies.

3. Infrastructure programs for poverty reduction

In addition to the construction of such infrastructure in poor villages as roads, water conservancy, drinking water, electricity and broadband, they also involve relocation of the poor people and renovation of dilapidated housing in rural areas. The government should speed up the relocation of impoverished rural populations from areas with harsh living conditions, fragile ecological environment and frequent natural disasters. It's planned to relocate 10 million poor people between 2016 and 2020 based on the development of new urbanization, small towns and industrial parks. The government and social funds should be pooled for rural development, such as transportation construction, farmland irrigation, land remediation, geological disaster prevention, and forestry ecology, in a bid to support the public facilities construction in the resettlement area and ecological restoration in the emigration areas. Support for housing construction, production and entrepreneurial discount loans should be provided for eligible relocated households.

4. Poverty reduction through ecological conservation

When it comes to major national ecological projects, preferences were given to poor areas in terms of the allocation of project and fund so as to involve and benefit more people in poverty. The government should step up efforts in ecological conservation and restoration in poverty-stricken areas, increase the transfer payment to key eco-function areas, create ecological jobs for the poor and increase ecological compensation.

5. Improve the care for left-behind children, women, elders and disabled people

The government should conduct thorough investigations into the left-behind children, women, elders and disabled people in rural China and establish a dynamic information system in this respect; enhance the building of facilities and capacities concerning children welfare homes, rescue and protection institutions, relief and support system for people in dire poverty, rehabilitation and care services for the disabled, and community-based children's home, while continuously improving the management and services. It should develop a system of care services for "left-behind" children featuring concerted efforts of families, schools, community-level Party organizations, governments and society; improve the guardianship of minors; perfect the welfare and service system for children in plight, including orphans, unaccompanied children, children from low-income families, and seriously ill or disabled children; step up efforts to implement projects for rehabilitation of the disabled, special education, skills training and foster services. Regarding the special difficulties of the disabled, it should establish a full-scale system of living subsidies for disabled persons with financial difficulties and nursing subsidies for persons with serious disabilities. For the key recipients of assistance, including the elders, minors and severely disabled people in rural families covered by the subsistence allowances, efforts should be made to improve the level of assistance to meet their basic needs in life. All sectors of society should be mobilized to participate in the care services for the special groups in need.

Furthermore, in a bid to solve the problem regional poverty, the Chinese government decided to continue to strengthen infrastructure construction in poverty-stricken areas to overcome obstacles to development. The main measures include accelerating the construction of facilities in transportation, water conservancy and electric power, intensifying efforts in "Internet Plus" model for poverty reduction, speeding up renovation of dilapidated housing in rural areas and improvement of rural living environment, with focus on the former revolutionary bases, areas inhabited by ethnic minorities, border areas and contiguous impoverished areas.

4.5.5 Establish Poverty Identification, Assistance, Assessment and Accountability Mechanisms

1. Establish the mechanism for accurate identification of poor population for poverty reduction

Since 2014, poverty archives or cards have been created for three types of groups for poverty reduction: impoverished households, villages and counties, with a nation-wide poverty reduction information system that's updated annually. The accurate identification of impoverished households is based on multidimensional indicators, covering income, education, health, housing and so on. China has two datasets of poverty monitoring and evaluation. One dataset shows the national poor population, incidence of poverty and distribution, prepared by the National Bureau of Statistics based on the household sample survey and national poverty line (determined by factoring both income and consumption). The other is about the information of the registered poor population, acquired by the State Council Leading Group Office of Poverty Alleviation and Development based on grassroots poverty identification and registration household by household. The criteria for poverty identification combine income with the multidimensional poverty indicators of adequate food and clothing and guaranteed access to education, basic medical service and housing, followed by policy and program support to the identified households.

2. Establish the mechanism of stationing officials in villages to work on poverty reduction

An assistance accountability mechanism tailored to each poor village and household has been put in place. In 2014, a total of 128,000 poverty-stricken villages were identified in the national survey. In line with the actual situation of these villages, one outstanding official was sent to each village as first secretary of the Party committee to build assistance work teams and cooperate with the CPC village committee and the villagers' committee to implement the measures for poverty reduction.[14] Given the causes of poverty and development needs, assistance plan was formulated to help poor villages and households with the implementation of poverty-reduction policies and programs and facilitate poverty eradication.

[14]Liu (2016).

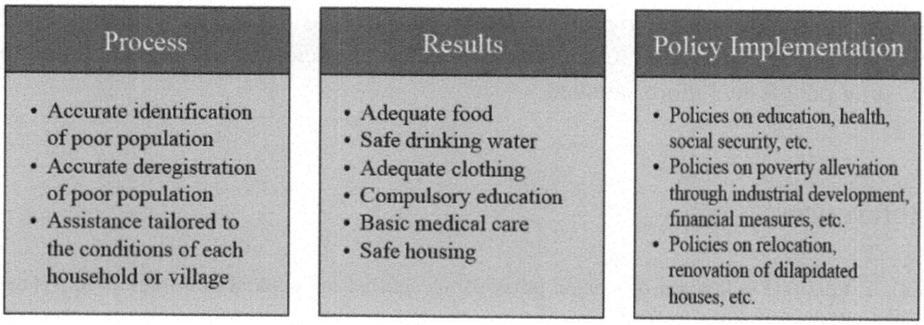

Fig. 4.5 Main contents for evaluation of poverty reduction achievements

3. Establish the performance evaluation mechanism for poverty reduction

From 2016 to 2020, an annual evaluation of the progress in poverty reduction by provincial Party committees and governments shall be conducted by the State Council Leading Group Office of Poverty Alleviation and Development, covering the progress in the annual poverty-reduction plan, the growth of government funds for poverty reduction, the per capita net income of farmers in poor areas, the accuracy in poverty identification and delisting, the poor people's satisfaction with the assistance programs, among others (see Fig. 4.5).[15]

4. Establish a third-party evaluation mechanism for poverty reduction achievements

With a view to evaluating the government's poverty reduction performance in an objective manner, a third-party agency conducts an independent evaluation on the provincial Party committees and governments on a yearly basis. The first third-party trial evaluation was implemented in 2016. In 2017, on the basis of summarizing the third-party trial evaluation, China officially launched a third-party evaluation in 22 provinces that signed to the letter of commitment on poverty elimination. What is under evaluation includes the progress toward the goal of adequate food and clothing and guaranteed access to education, basic medical service and housing, accuracy in poverty identification and delisting, as well as the people's satisfaction with the poverty reduction work. The third-party evaluation remains independent, objective, fair and scientific in order to ensure the authenticity of the results.

5. Establish the accountability mechanism

Based on the results from the above third-party evaluations, the State Council Leading Group Office of Poverty Alleviation and Development would conduct an interview with the heads of provincial Party committees and governments that lag behind in poverty reduction and demand rectifications accordingly. In this way, the evaluation and accountability mechanisms play a role of "baton" to direct and urge the officials

[15] General Office of the CPC Central Committee and General Office of the State Council (2016).

in poor areas to prioritize poverty reduction, and strive to achieve the goal of poverty elimination by 2020, build a moderately prosperous society in all respect, and help the poor people feel more satisfied.

References

Gao, T. (2014). Declaration of war on poverty: Specialized agricultural construction in "Three Western Areas." *Ningxia Times*.

General Office of the CPC Central Committee and General Office of the State Council. (2016). Procedures for Performance Evaluation of the Provincial Party Committees and Governments in Poverty Alleviation and Development. Website of the State Council. http://www.gov.cn.

General Office of the State Council. (1986). Notice on the Establishment of the State Council Leading Group of Economic Development in Poor Areas (Guo Ban Fa [1986] No.39). Website of the central government. http://www.gov.cn.

General Office of the State Council. (1988). Notice on Reorganizing the State Council Leading Group of Economic Development in Poor Areas (Guo Ban Fa [1988] No.30). Website of the central government. http://www.gov.cn.

Information Office of the State Council. (2011). New Progress in Development-oriented Poverty Reduction Program for Rural China.

Liu, Y. (2016). Make targeted efforts to improve the results of fight against poverty. *People's Daily*.

Notice of the State Council on Promulgation of the National Plan for Poverty Alleviation in the 13th Five-Year Plan Period. (November 2016). Guo Fa [2016] No.64. Website of the State Council Leading Group Office of Poverty Alleviation and Development. http://www.cpad.gov.cn.

The Decision of the CPC Central Committee and the State Council on Eradicating Poverty in China (Zhong Fa (2015) No.34). (November 29, 2015). Website of the State Council Leading Group Office of Poverty Alleviation and Development. http://www.cpad.gov.cn.

Wang, X. (2012). *The measurement of poverty: Theories and methods* (2nd ed.), Social Sciences Academic Press.

Zhang, L. (2007a). *The course of poverty reduction in China (1949–2005)*, China Financial and Economic Publishing House.

Zhang, L. (2007b). *The evolution of poverty reduction policies in China (1949–2005)*, China Financial and Economic Publishing House.

Chapter 5
System of Development-Oriented Poverty-Reduction Policies in China

China's policy system for poverty reduction incorporates economic policies on pro-poor growth, social policies to narrow the income gap and promote social equity, as well as special poverty-reduction policies targeting poor areas and poor people. This chapter successively reviews and evaluates China's economic policies on pro-poor growth, social policies to promote inclusive development and special poverty-reduction polices, before introducing China's policy system on poverty reduction during the 13th Five-Year Plan period (2016–2020).

5.1 Pro-poor Economic Growth Policies

5.1.1 Is China's Economic Growth Pro-poor?

Sustained economic growth is the foundation for poverty eradication. Whether the economic growth is a boon for poverty reduction depends on the possibility for the poor people to actively participate in and significantly benefit from economic activity. According to the theory of trickle-down development, the benefits of economic growth go to the rich first, and then in the second round the poor begin to benefit when the rich start spending their gains. Thus, the poor benefit from economic growth only indirectly through a vertical flow from the rich. It implies that the proportional benefits of growth going to the poor will always be less. In fact, as the income is distributed less fairly, it's possible that the economic growth increases poverty. This also goes some way toward explaining the unmatched progress in poverty reduction with the sustained economic growth in some countries.

X. Wang and X. Zhang, *Towards 2030 – China's Poverty Alleviation and Global Poverty Governance*, International Research on Poverty Reduction,
https://doi.org/10.1007/978-981-15-6356-0_5

It raises the question: is China's economic growth pro-poor? This chapter will answer the question based on the Pro-poor Growth Index (PPGI) developed by Kakwani and Permia.[1]

To understand, therefore, the impact of economic growth on poverty, one needs to measure separately the impact of changes in average income and those in its distribution. In other words, one needs to break down the total change in poverty into (i) the impact of growth when the distribution of income does not change, and (ii) the effect of income redistribution when total income does not change.

Suppose O is the proportional change in poverty when there a positive growth rate of one percent. This can be broken down into two components, O_g and O_I such that

$$O = O_g + O_I$$

where O_g is the pure growth effect and O_I is the inequality effect. O_g is the percentage change in poverty when the distribution of income does not change, whereas O_I is the change in poverty when inequality changes in the absence of growth.

Suppose θ is a poverty measure that is fully characterized by the poverty line income, then

$$\theta = \theta\,(\mathrm{z},\ \mu,\ L(p))$$

where z is the poverty line, μ is the mean income of the society and $L(p)$ the Lorenz function, which is interpreted as the percentage share of income enjoyed by the bottom p percent of the population. The total proportional change in poverty between period 1 and 2 as P_{12} can be interpreted as:

$$P_{12} = \ln\{\theta[z, \mu_2, L_2(p)]\} - \ln\{\theta[z, \mu_1, L_1(p)]\}$$

where μ_1 and μ_2 are the mean incomes in years 1 and 2, respectively, and $L_1(p)$ and $L_2(p)$ are the Lorenz curves for years 1 and 2, respectively. Note that mean incomes μ_1 and μ_2 are adjusted for price changes between the two periods but the poverty line is fixed in each period.

The pure growth effect is defined as the proportional change in poverty when the mean income changes but the relative income distribution measured by the Lorenz curve remains unchanged. Similarly, the pure inequality effect is defined as the change in poverty when the Lorenz curve changes but the mean income at constant prices remains constant.

Let us denote the growth effect by G_{12} and the inequality effect by I_{12} between years 1 and 2. Then, the change in poverty can be expressed as:

$$P_{12} = f\,(G_{12},\ I_{12})$$

[1] Kakwani and Permia (2000).

Suppose that there is a positive growth rate of g_{12} percent between periods 1 and 2, then poverty elasticity can be defined as

$$\eta = P_{12}/g_{12}$$

which is the proportional change in total poverty when there is a positive growth rate of 1 percent. Likewise, we may define

$$\eta_g = G_{12}/g_{12}$$

$$\eta_I = I_{12}/g_{12}$$

where η_g is the proportional change in poverty when there is a positive growth rate of 1% provided the relative inequality does not change, that is, pure growth effect in poverty; whereas η_I is the proportional change in poverty when inequality changes but the real mean income does not change, which is pure distribution effect in poverty. It means:

$$\eta = \eta_g + \eta_I$$

which shows that the proportional change in poverty caused by a 1% positive growth rate in the economy is the sum of the two factors: η_g is the income effect of growth on poverty and η_I is the inequality effect on poverty.

The income effect of growth on poverty, η_g, is always negative, which implies that growth will always reduce poverty when the relative inequality does not change. The inequality effect, ηI, can be either negative or positive. If η_I is negative, it means that growth has led to a change in the distribution of income in favor of the poor, thereby reducing poverty unequivocally. Such growth can be characterized as pro-poor. If η_I is positive, the change in income distribution is pro-rich. This suggests that we can have an index of pro-poor growth

$$\varphi = \eta_I/\eta_g$$

φ will be greater than 1 if $\eta_I < 0$, which means that growth is strictly pro-poor. If $0 < \varphi < 1$, it means that $\eta_I > 0$ but poverty still declines due to growth. This situation may be generally characterized as trickle-down. If $\varphi < 0$, economic growth in fact badly hurts the poor and leads to an increase in poverty.

The disadvantage of this approach is that it doesn't factor in the level of real growth, even though it considered whether the poor could benefit from changes in income distribution. Furthermore, the approach doesn't take monotonicity axiom into consideration.

Following the above approach, this chapter measures the pro-poor growth in China based on the data of China Health and Nutrition Survey from 1989 to 2009. The

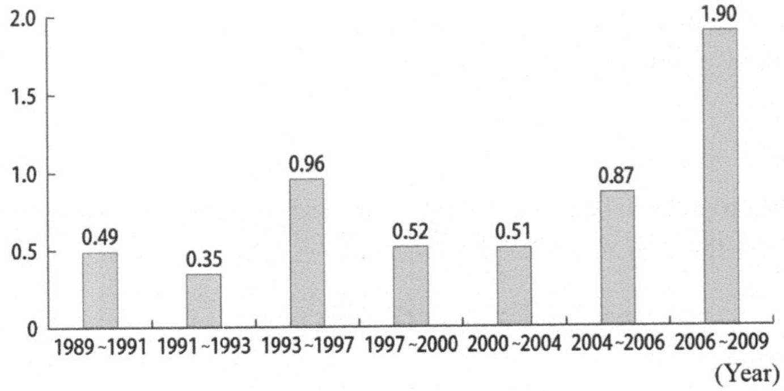

Fig. 5.1 Measurement of Kakwani and Pernia's PPGI

dataset covers nine surveyed provinces of Liaoning, Heilongjiang, Jiangsu, Shandong, Henan, Hubei, Hunan, Guangxi and Guizhou in eight years: 1989, 1991, 1993, 1997, 2000, 2004, 2006 and 2009. Figure 5.1 shows the measurement of PPGI.

We can clearly see that during the six different growth periods between 1989 and 2006, the PPGI varied between 0 and 1, indicating that economic growth reduces poverty, but not strictly pro-poor. The poverty reduction mainly comes from trickle-down development. The PPGI between 2006 and 2009 was 1.90, greater than 1, indicating that the economic growth is strictly pro-poor.[2]

5.1.2 Policies Conducive to Pro-poor Growth in China

Looking back at the economic policies since the 1980s, the most important policies to promote China's large-scale poverty reduction relate to the following three fields: land reform, rural workforce transfer and universal access to infrastructure. The policies concerning the first two fields are important public policies to release the vitality of production factors and increase productivity, while universal access to infrastructure fosters China's industrialization, urbanization and sustained high-speed growth, and thus laying a solid foundation for large-scale poverty reduction.

1. Land reform

Around the 1980s, China implemented the household contract responsibility system of rural land, allowing farmers to contract a portion of the collectively owned land and enjoy the right to land use and earnings. The policy was later introduced to extend the second-round rural land contracts by another 30 years upon their expiration. Given that the arable land per person in China is less than 0.1 hectare, the above land policy makes it possible for each rural household to have a share of arable

[2]For more details, please refer to Chap. 12 of the book *The Measurement of Poverty: Theories and Methods* by Wang Xiaolin published by Social Sciences Academic Press in 2017.

land. In addition, they have the right to claim surplus earnings from their agricultural operations. Amartya Sen believes that the most important means to eradicate hunger and poverty is the production-based entitlement. Land property rights in developed countries are usually complete and clearly defined, but not necessarily fair. China's land policy may mark the first time in human history to give the most equitable land use rights to every household. This is the most important entitlement to production.

Thanks to the above system, China's agricultural output registered an annual growth of 9% on average from 1979 to 1984. Based on an agricultural production function analysis, Justin Lin Yifu estimated that the household contract responsibility system led to an increase of 46–89% in agricultural output from 1978 to 1984.[3] The per capita net income of farmers increased from RMB 133.6 in 1978 to RMB 397.6 in 1985; the rural poor population fell from 250 million in 1978 to 125 million in 1985, accompanied by the drop in the incidence of poverty from 30.7 to 14.8%.[4] Over seven years, the net income of farmers increased by 197.6%, the rural population down by 50% and the incidence of poverty down by 15.9%. This should be mainly contributed to the institutional and policy reforms.

In countries with a relatively large poor population, such as India and Bangladesh, and countries with relatively high Gini coefficients, such as most countries in Latin America, the farmers' unfair access to land has been the main institutional obstacle for growth conducive to poverty reduction.

2. Rural workforce transfer

Wage raise for rural workers who migrate to urban areas for work in non-agricultural sectors, such as industrial and service sectors has been a major driver for poverty reduction. In the early and mid-1990s, with the abolition of the food rationing system, rural laborers were allowed to go for urban employment. In the Yangtze River Delta and the Pearl River Delta particularly, the development of export-oriented and labor-intensive processing industries absorbed a large pool of rural laborers. The free flow of population, especially the rural population, as the most important production factor, is another important contributor to the large-scale poverty reduction in China. Despite China's household registration system that resulted in the unequal access to public services for urban and rural residents, the large-scale migration of rural people to work in non-agricultural sectors in urban areas is unstoppable. The rural workforce transfer has been another important pillar for China's industrialization and urbanization, as well as the foundation for massive poverty reduction in rural areas.

Since the early 1980s, the size of the floating population has begun to expand rapidly. In 1982, the floating population stood at merely 6.57 million, and that number has continued to rise in the twenty-first century. In accordance with the Communiqué on Major Data of 1% National Population Sample Survey in 2005, as of 0:00 a.m. November 1, 2005, the national floating population reached 147.35 million, accounting for more than 11% of the country's total population. According to the Statistical Communiqué of the People's Republic of China on the 2015 National

[3]Lin (1994).

[4]The data are derived from *China Statistical Yearbook* compiled by the National Statistics Bureau.

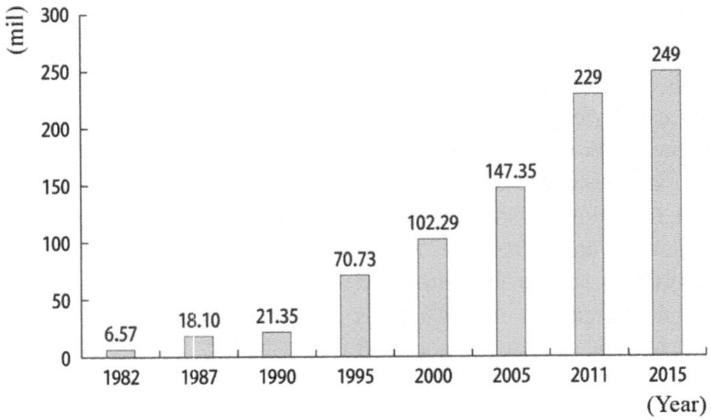

Fig. 5.2 China's floating population. *Source* The 1982, 1990, 1995, 2000 data is from census data, 1987 and 2005 data from 1% population sample survey, 2011 data from China Migrants Dynamic Survey 2011, and 2015 data from Statistical Communiqué of the People's Republic of China on the 2015 National Economic and Social Development

Economic and Social Development, the floating population by 2015 reached 249 million, making up 18% of the total population. About 80% of the floating population was rural-to-urban migrants and the remaining 20% urban-to-urban migrants. By 2015, the number of rural workers in non-agricultural employment was 277.47 million, including 168.84 million migrant workers and 108.63 million local rural workers, making up 60.8 and 39.2% of the total number of rural workers, respectively (see Fig. 5.2).

With the population movement and the transfer of rural workforce to non-agricultural sectors, the income structure has changed significantly with the rapid increase in the per capita net income of farmers. In 1990, the per capita net income of farmers reached RMB 686, of which wage income only accounted for 20.2%; by 2013, the amount increased to RMB 8,896, of which wage income made up 45.2%.

3. Universal access to infrastructure

It goes without saying that China's poverty reduction has benefited from sustained rapid economic growth for more than 30 years. However, a basic condition for the transformation of labor advantage into comparative advantages in manufacturing industry lies in the construction of appropriate infrastructure, so as to reduce logistics costs and turn resource advantages into competitive edge in market. As a popular saying in rural China says, transportation infrastructure is fundamental for a region's development. In other words, infrastructure development is more a public consensus than a government will.

In 2015, China's total road mileage reached 4.5 million km, including 108,000 km of expressways. The 13th Five-Year Plan made it clear to further strengthen the construction of transportation infrastructure. In the poorest Guizhou Province in southwestern China, all counties had been connected by expressways as of 2015.

Currently, China boasts over 20,000 km of high-speed railways, ranking first in the world. During the 13th Five-Year Plan period, the high-speed railways will extend at an annual rate of over 50%. As the world's largest producer of renewable energy, China's priority in the hydropower development has been well recognized by the international community. In 2015, global hydropower capacity was 1,212 GW, of which China accounted for 27%.[5] The universal access to electricity plays an extremely important role in promoting pro-poor growth and eradicating extreme poverty. See Box 5.1 for the hydropower development in China.

Box 5.1 Hydropower development in China

In 2015, the total installed hydropower capacity in China reached 319 million kW, making up one quarter of the world's total. During the 12th Five-Year Plan period, the newly installed capacity of conventional hydropower was approximately 98 million kW, bringing the total installed capacity to 297 million kW by the end of 2015, with a completion rate of 115%. The power generation exceeded the planned target as well, reaching 1.1 trillion kWh and making up 19.9% of the national power generation and 73.9% of the non-fossil energy. It is estimated that by 2020, the installed capacity of conventional hydropower in China will reach 340 million kW, that of pumped storage power stations 45 million kW and that of hydropower about 380 million kW.

Source China Statistical Yearbook and *Hydropower Status Report 2016.*

5.2 Social Policies that Facilitate Inclusive Development

The policies in education, health and social security play an important role in securing the people's basic livelihoods, preventing the intergenerational transmission of poverty, creating fair development opportunities to prevent the poor from losing from the beginning, and promoting social inclusion and equity. China is committed to building a more equitable and universally accessible social policy system that will significantly contribute to poverty eradication.

Inclusive development puts more emphasis on the fairness at the starting point. To quote from Chinese government officials, "Don't let the poor lose at the starting line," highlighting equal opportunities. In the latest round of the fight against poverty (2016–2020), one of the overall goals of development-oriented poverty reduction is to achieve indices of major basic public services close to the national average levels. This is a basic requirement for the transformation of social development.

[5] IHA (2016).

5.2.1 Policies for Poverty Reduction Through Education

The Chinese government has long implemented the poverty-reduction policies on preferential education targeting poor areas and poor people, in a bid to promote balanced development of education and creating more equitable development opportunities. The policies for poverty reduction through education in recent years mainly fall into the following categories.

1. Policies to improve school conditions

In response to schools at different stages of education, *the Action Plan for Three-Year Preschool Education* was launched and the conditions of disadvantaged schools of compulsory education in poverty-ridden areas were improved overall.

A. *The Action Plan for Three-Year Preschool Education*

Preschool education marks the beginning of lifelong learning. It is an essential part of the national education system, an important social welfare undertaking, as well as the foundation to block the intergenerational transmission of poverty and promote social equity. China has made nine-year compulsory education universally accessible, but preschool education is still underdeveloped across the country, evidenced by the shortage of educational resources, investment and teachers, inadequate institutions and rules, urban–rural disparity, and more notably, poor access for children in poverty-stricken areas. In response, *the Action Plan for Three-Year Preschool Education* was initiated and the first three-year phase began in 2011. All-out efforts were made to build public kindergartens and provide public services in preschool education featuring "wide coverage and guarantee of basic needs." More government funds were earmarked to build, renovate and expand a large number of safe and applicable kindergartners. All sectors of the society were mobilized to build kindergartens in various forms with the support of a series of measures, including reasonable land use and tax breaks. Active support was provided for the development of private kindergartens, especially those inclusive and low-cost ones. Efforts were made to enrich resources for preschool education and accelerate the development of kindergartens by incorporating it into the plan for public service facilities in new rural areas. Thanks to the implementation of the action plan in numerous counties as well as eight major national programs in preschool education since 2011, the number of enrolled children in kindergartens increased 9.18 million in three years, while the three-year preschool gross enrollment rate reached 67.5%, up by 10.9% in three years. These are historic achievements arising from the reform and development of preschool education.[6] In 2014, China launched the second three-year phase of the action plan (2014–2016), with the goal to increase the three-year preschool gross enrollment rate to 75% by 2016.[7]

---

[6]Opinions of the State Council on Current Development of Preschool Education (2010).

[7]The Interpretation of Ministry of Education on the Opinions on Implementing the Second Action Plan for Three-Year Preschool Education. http://www.gov.cn/xinwen/2014-11/16/content2779388.htm.

B. The conditions of disadvantaged schools of compulsory education in poverty-ridden areas were improved overall. Despite the remarkable achievements in popularizing compulsory education, there has been a rising call for balanced urban–rural and inter-regional development of education. In particular, due to the backward socioeconomic development in rural, remote, impoverished and ethnic minority areas, the cost of running schools and learning centers is higher, teaching conditions poorer, and facilities like dormitories and canteens insufficient. In such context, it's difficult to run village primary schools, the teachers are not enough and the dropout rate is higher, making it a weak link of compulsory education in China. To solve these problems, China began to improve the basic conditions of disadvantaged schools of compulsory education in poverty-ridden areas from 2013.[8] The program focuses on improving the basic facilities of compulsory education in 832 poverty-stricken counties, involving classroom renovation for rural junior high schools, building rural boarding schools, and full coverage of digital educational resources for learning centers in villages. The main goal is that in three to five years, schools of compulsory education in poor areas shall be equipped with basic teaching facilities, including classrooms, tables and chairs, books, laboratory instruments, and sports grounds, as well as basic living facilities, such as dormitories, beds, toilets, canteens and access to safe drinking water; the basic learning and boarding needs of the left-behind children shall be satisfied; the village primary schools and learning centers shall run smoothly; the super-large size of classes in counties shall be reduced to no more than 45 students in one class in primary schools and no more than 50 in junior high schools; the teachers shall be allocated more rationally, with the quantity, quality and structure befitting the basic teaching needs; the dropout rate in primary schools shall be controlled below 0.6%, and that in junior high school below 1.8%.

2. Policies to improve student nutrition

Since 2011, China has begun to offer a nutritious mean allowance of RMB 3 (raised to RMB 4 in November 2014) per day per student receiving compulsory education in contiguous impoverished areas, benefiting 32.1 million rural students as of June 2015. The monitoring results show the improvement to various degrees in terms of the average height, weight and academic scores of male and female students aged 6–15 in poverty-stricken areas.[9]

3. Policies to reduce student spending

First, the policy to waive tuition and miscellaneous fees, supply free textbooks and grant living allowances for rural boarders receiving compulsory education from poor families. Free textbooks are provided to rural students and students from urban families covered by subsistence allowances. Rural students are provided with free Chinese

[8]According to the Opinions on Overall Improvement of Basic Conditions of Disadvantaged Schools of Compulsory Education in Poverty-ridden Areas [Department of Basic Education, Ministry of Education. (2013) No.10].

[9]China's Implementation of 20 Poverty Alleviation Policies through Education towards Full Coverage of Poor Areas. Xinhuanet. October 15, 2015.

dictionaries as well. The living allowances are granted to rural and urban students from financially disadvantaged families receiving compulsory education. Students in primary schools and junior high schools in central and western China are entitled to a living allowance of RMB 4 and RMB 5 per day, respectively. Second, the policy to fund the regular senior high school students. In 2010, China introduced the policy to offer state grants for regular senior high school students from families in financial difficulties, which averages RMB 2,000 for each recipient annually, covering 20% of the students. In 2014 alone, 4.95 million students received from the grants. Third, the policy to exempt tuition fees and allot living subsidies to students at secondary vocational schools. Starting from the fall semester in 2012, a tuition fee waiver program in secondary vocational schools, under which the tuition fees based on a standard of RMB 2,000 per student per year for all rural students (including the ones from counties and towns), urban students who major in agriculture and those poverty-stricken students at full-time secondary vocational schools were abolished. State grants at the standard of RMB 2000 per student per year are also given to full-time first and second-year students majoring in agriculture and those non-agriculture majors from poverty-stricken families, covering 100% of students from contiguous impoverished areas. Fourth, the policy to fund students receiving higher education. Currently, such policies integrate national scholarship, national encouragement scholarship, state grants, state-subsidized student loans, free tuition for normal university students, work-study programs, tuition waivers, "express channel" and other forms of assistances.[10]

4. Policies to improve teachers' quality

The *Rural Teacher Support Program (2015–2020)* is implemented to build a team of high-quality and dedicated teachers stationed in rural areas, by means of expanding channels to recruit rural teachers, improving the living conditions, among others.

5. Special policies for regions inhabited by ethnic minority groups

First, extend the years of free education in regions inhabited by ethnic minority groups, such as 15-year free education in Tibet, 14-year free education in the four prefectures in southern Xinjiang (Hotan, Aksu and Kashi prefectures, and Kizilsu Kirgiz autonomous prefecture) and 12-year free education (covering nine-year compulsory education and three-year high school education) in Tibetan-inhabited areas of Sichuan Province. Second, special polices were formulated to support education in Tibet and Xinjiang. As of 2014, 19 provinces and municipalities that provide aid to Xinjiang had carried out 386 education programs, invested RMB 8.5 billion, trained 140,000 teachers and sent over 3,000 volunteers to teach in rural areas. Third, since 2012, the mechanism for pair-up assistance between 10 vocational education groups in the developed regions in eastern China and 17 prefectures in Tibet and Tibetan-inhabited areas of Sichuan Province. Fourth, provide pair-up assistance to colleges and universities in Xinjiang and Tibet. Since 2010, the Ministry of Education

[10]China's Implementation of 20 Poverty Alleviation Policies through Education towards Full Coverage of Poor Areas. Xinhuanet. October 15, 2015.

has established six teams to provide pair-up assistance to 42 colleges and universities in Xinjiang and Tibet. Fifth, open special classes of junior and senior high school education and vocational education for students from Tibet and Xinjiang in the inner land, organize preparatory classes for students of ethnic minorities and initiated high-level personnel training programs for ethnic minorities.

5.2.2 Policies for Poverty Reduction Through Health Promotion

Since the launch of development-oriented poverty-reduction program in an organized and planned way in 1986, China's national health has made substantial progress. By 2015, the under-five mortality rate dropped to 11‰ and the maternal mortality rate down to 2.7‰. [11]

In response to the rising percentage of families caught in or sent back to poverty due to illness, difficult access to and expensive medical treatment, and other serious problems, the Chinese government designated key regions, key groups of people and major diseases for support during the 13th Five-Year Plan period. To this end, it's proposed to further strengthen overall planning and coordination and integrate resources, take effective measures to improve the medical services for the rural poor population and in poverty-stricken regions, improve the health of rural poor people in an all-round way and provide health guarantee for the rural poor people as they join the nation in building a moderately prosperous society in all aspects. A mechanism connecting basic medical insurance, serious disease insurance with medical assistance should be set up to play a synergistic and complementary role in providing medical services for the poor in an all-round way (see Fig. 5.3).

1. Basic medical insurance

By 2015, the New Rural Cooperative Medical System (NRCMS) had covered over 97% of rural residents. The NRCMS offers a per capita subsidy of RMB 380 and reimbursement ratios of outpatient and inpatient costs reached 50 and 75%.[12] But for the poor people, the remaining 25% out-of-pocket payment for inpatient treatment is still too expensive to afford. In this context, the fee to join the NRCMS for the registered poor population is subsidized by the government and reimbursement rates for inpatient costs are raised. To address the problems in coordinated hospitalization for serious diseases and low reimbursement rate of outpatient costs, local governments have explored a compensation mechanism for high outpatient costs. For example, Shanxi Province includes high blood pressure, diabetes, and other 33

[11] World Bank (2016). In 2016, the average life expectancy reached 76.34 in China. The Statistical Communiqué of the People's Republic of China on the 2015 National Economic and Social Development (2016a).

[12] National Health and Family Planning Commission (2016b).

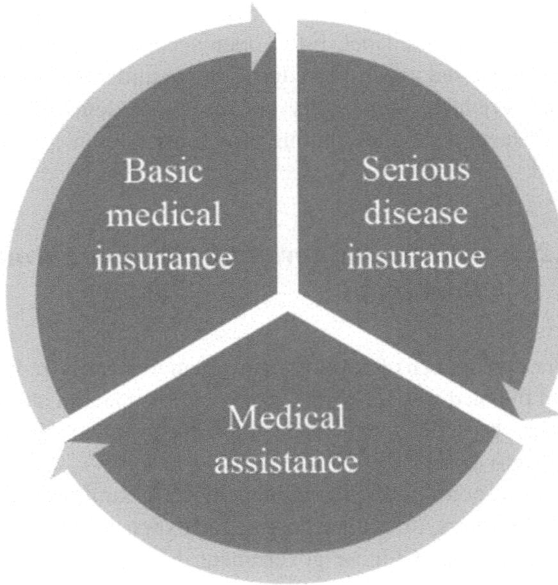

Fig. 5.3 China's medical insurance system

chronic and recurrent diseases that require no inpatient treatments into NRCMS, raising the compensation rate to 60–80%.

2. Serious disease insurance

Serious illness insurance for urban and rural residents has been fully implemented, lowering the deductible line while raising the reimbursement rate. The treatment-before-payment policy has been carried out for inpatient treatment of rural poor people in counties. For instance, in 2016, Shanxi Province lowered the deductible line for serious disease insurance from RMB 10,000 to RMB 5,000 and raised the actual reimburse rate of serious disease insurance by two to three percentage points, with the maximum compensation at RMB 400,000. Moreover, the province raised the reimbursement rate of inpatient costs to 70% for 24 serious diseases, including malignant tumors, uremia, congenital heart disease of children and leukemia, with 20% from government assistance and the remaining 10% paid by the patients.

3. Medical assistance

Universal medical assistance shall be provided to all rural poor people suffering from major diseases to reduce their medical burden. For the patients who get seriously ill and cannot get family support in time, more temporary assistance shall be provided and active efforts shall be made to seek help from charity organizations.

In addition to the above three key medical insurances, efforts shall be made to train more doctors in poor rural areas, build village clinics, improve the public health services as well as maternal and child healthcare services, take advantage of low-cost traditional Chinese medicine, and improve the diagnosis and treatment capabilities of hospitals in poor areas through telemedicine.

5.2.3 Social Security Policies

It's proposed to "establish the system of subsistence allowance in rural areas in due course" at the Sixth Plenary Session of the 16th CPC Central Committee in 2006. The *Notice of the State Council on Establishing the System of Subsistence Allowance throughout Rural China* was promulgated in 2007. The goal of the system is to cover all eligible rural poor people and ensure adequate food and clothing for the rural poor in a stable, sustained and effective way. The standards of rural subsistence allowance are determined by local governments above the county level on the basis of the fees needed for such basic necessities as food, clothing, water, electricity and other things throughout the year. The standards shall be reported to the people's government at a higher level for registration before being published and implemented. Such standards shall be adjusted timely in line with the rising price of local necessities and the people's living standards. The subsistence allowance system covers all rural residents whose per-capita annual net household income was below the prescribed standard, as well as the rural residents suffering from perennial difficulties due to illness, disability, old age, poor health, incapability for work and harsh living conditions. Currently, China's rural poverty-reduction landscape mainly features the development-oriented poverty-reduction system and the subsistence allowance system.

Each system has developed its own characteristics in practice. The development-oriented poverty-reduction system mainly targets the poor people with working ability. It aims to create better conditions for the development of the poor people by improving the production conditions in these areas (mainly counties and villages), particularly the infrastructure and public services. It aims to help the poor get rid of poverty by developing their capabilities for production and employment. On the other hand, the subsistence allowance system mainly targets the poor people without working ability and aims to meet their basic needs with assistance in cash.

As shown in Fig. 5.4, as of the end of 2015, the subsistence allowance system covered 28.462 million rural households, totaling 49.036 million people. The subsidy funds from governments at all levels for rural subsistence allowances reached RMB 93.15 billion. The average standard was RMB 3,177.6 per person per year in 2015, up by 14.4% over the previous year. The average subsidy was RMB 1,766.5 per person per year, up by 13.8% from the previous year.[13]

A survey by Huawei Han and Yuebin Xu based on large samples of households in five provinces in central and western China showed that the rural subsistence allowance system reduced the poverty among the sampled subjects significantly. Factors that matters most for its anti-poverty effect include the system's coverage,

[13]Ministry of Civil Affairs (2016).

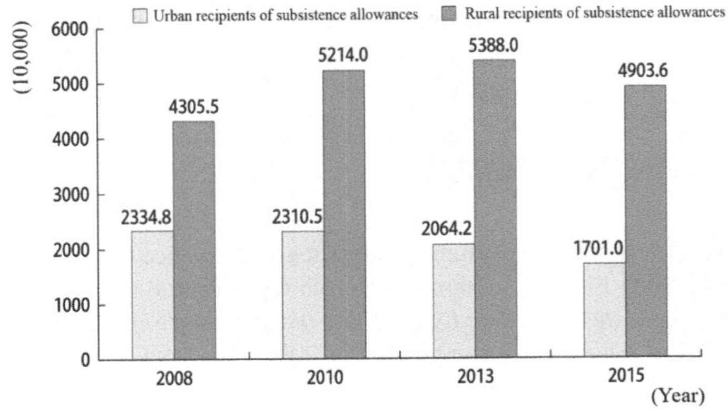

Fig. 5.4 Number of urban and rural recipients of subsistence allowances. *Source* Ministry of Civil Affairs (2016)

accuracy of the targets and standard of the subsistence allowance. The funds for rural subsistence allowances are mainly raised by local governments and the financially challenged areas shall be subsidized by the central government. Due to the backward economic development in central and western regions, the local government is in serious financial difficulties. Against the backdrop of limited transfer payment from the central government, many poor areas adopted the strategy of "offering subsistence allowances based on the local financial capacity."[14] In this context, low coverage and standard of subsistence allowances constitute two key factors that negatively affect the anti-poverty effect. Furthermore, the poor accuracy in targeting the recipients also undermined the system's effect on poverty reduction.

At present, the central government has put forward the goal of eradicating poverty by 2020, measured as the current poverty line, while requiring the rural subsistence allowance system to help the most impoverished people get rid of poverty. To this end, the rural subsistence allowance standard should be raised above the national poverty line, while ensuring the accuracy in identifying the recipients. Given the great difficulty in accurately calculating the farmers' income, the identification of recipients should factor in both income and non-income elements.

5.3 Anti-poverty Projects and Initiatives

Based on the definition of multidimensional poverty and under the guidance of cross-department leading groups of development-oriented poverty reduction, a "three-in-one" poverty-reduction system has taken shape, integrating special poverty-reduction programs, poverty reduction through industrial development and social

[14]Han and Xu (2014).

involvement in poverty reduction. Special poverty-reduction programs refer to the programs specially devised for poverty-stricken areas and people, incorporating relocation program, integrated village development, work relief, poverty reduction through industrial development, employment promotion, pilot poverty-reduction programs, Dewdrop program, among others. The development-oriented poverty-reduction offices set by governments at all levels are put in charge for the implementation of these programs. The government bodies in charge of agriculture, education, health, transportation and other areas shall formulate and carry out their respective poverty-reduction policies. The policies for social involvement in poverty reduction aim to mobilize the participation of all social sectors. Since the establishment of a special department for development-oriented poverty reduction in 1986, a slew of policies for special poverty-reduction programs have been devised. The following section shall analyze such policies from the perspective of the government funding for poverty reduction, including the funds appropriated by the central government and local supporting funds.

5.3.1 Work Relief Programs

Under the work relief program, the government invests in public infrastructure construction, offering opportunities for the poverty-stricken people to work for money, instead of offering direct relief. The work relief program is an important part of the poverty-reduction policies in rural China, allowing the local poor farmers to participate in the infrastructure construction in exchange for labor remuneration and increase their income directly. The government investment could be made in capital or in-kind and shall be accounted for in the form of the capital converted from in-kind. The government funding for work relief programs shall be sourced from poverty-reduction funds within the central government budget and investment of the central budget. The local investment in the work relief program shall be incorporated into the fiscal budget of the local government.

The work relief programs focus on the construction of rural small- and medium-scale infrastructure projects that promote the economic development in poverty-stricken regions and help farmers get rid of poverty and achieve prosperity, including the construction of basic farmland, works of farmland irrigation, roads (including standalone bridges and culverts) in counties, grassland construction, comprehensive improvement of small river basins, comprehensive regional development and other programs required by the state.[15] See Box 5.2 for "work relief" programs with the input of industrial goods coupons.

[15]National Development and Reform Commission (2014).

Box 5.2 Work relief in the form of industrial goods coupons

Between 1984 and 1987, China carried out the work relief program with the input of grain, cotton and cloth in 25 provinces and regions to build roads, waterways and small-scale water conservancy projects in poverty-stricken areas.

The program focused on 18 contiguous poverty-stricken areas. In 1987, the pilot work relief program with the input of medium- and low-grade industrial goods was launched in Sichuan Province, Jiangxi Province and Ningxia Hui Autonomous Region, for the purpose of building roads and water conservancy projects in poor areas. The workers could receive labor remuneration in the form of industrial goods or the coupons for industrial goods. After 2000, such labor remuneration was mostly paid in cash.

Source Compiled by the author based on the historical data relating to development-oriented poverty reduction in China, 2016

5.3.2 Policies to Support the Development in Economically Underdeveloped Areas

In 1986, China promulgated the policy of development funds for the economically underdeveloped areas (hereinafter referred to as "development funds"). This policy and the special funds originally targeted at improving the production conditions for agriculture and animal husbandry in poor areas, developing a diversified economy and promoting the development of commodity economy in rural China. The funds were mainly distributed to collective economy and poor households. The Administrative Provisions for Government Funds for Poverty Reduction (Trial) issued in 2000 further clarify that the funds shall be mainly used for the development of farm production and animal farming as well as the poverty reduction through science and technology (such as the introduction of superior crop varieties, the promotion of and training on advanced and practical technologies), while being appropriately used to build rural roads and villages, basic farmland (including grassland, orchids and forests), and farmland water conservancy projects, provide safe drinking water for people and livestock, and develop basic education, medical care, culture, radio and TV access, among others. With the changes in the distribution of poor population, the development policies that had mainly targeted at certain areas gradually evolved to the poverty-reduction policies targeting at both areas and households. Following the introduction of a host of innovative poverty-reduction policies since 2013, a full-fledged policy system in support of the poor people's development has been put in place, incorporating poverty reduction through industrial development, e-commerce and photovoltaic power generation, Dewdrop Project (to provide vocational training for the laborers from poor households), and so on.

Case No. 1 Poverty reduction through industrial development

In 2013, the State Council Leading Group Office of Poverty Alleviation and Development set up pilot reform zones for poverty reduction, allowing the developed areas to explore new mechanisms and models for poverty reduction. As one of the most developed provinces in China, Zhejiang explored a relatively successful model for poverty reduction through industrial development. Longquan City in the province prioritized the development of black fungus as the key agricultural industry with local characteristics and established a model of "company + specialized cooperative + base farmers." In 2013, the city's total agricultural output reached RMB 1.949 billion, with one-third from the black fungus industry which also created one-third of the jobs and income for farmers. Zhejiang Tianhe Food Co., Ltd. has been a leading company in the black fungus industry as well as in national poverty reduction. In 2013, the company's output value reached RMB 104 million, ranking the third in China in terms of the self-export of edible fungus. The company developed a standardized base covering an area of 1,600μ (about 106.67 hectares) employing 500 rural households, as well as an area of 3,200μ for order production that engaged 15,000 rural households.

Source The survey of the author in April 2014.

Case No. 2 Tibet's exploration of "Internet + targeted poverty reduction"

E-commerce for poverty reduction is an effective way to use mobile Internet technology to promote the development of agricultural products and services in poverty-stricken areas. The booming "Internet +" technology in China has opened up a new channel for development-oriented poverty reduction. Tibet is the dream destination for travelers, explorers and photographers alike, as well as the home to a wealth of tourism resources. Compared with the secondary industry, the tourism and service industry offers a greener and more sustainable way of poverty reduction, echoing the development vision advocated by the Chinese government in the 13th Five-Year Plan, and marking one of the concrete steps toward the UN's Sustainable Development Goals by 2030.

In 2015, the Tibet Autonomous Region invested RMB 18.5 million in each of the four counties it selected for implementing the pilot program of e-commerce for poverty reduction, with the focus on the development of the "Internet + tourism + special agricultural products" model. Under the program, the e-commerce companies provide development ideas and marketing methods, tourism companies take responsibility for operations and creating the travel experience, the government provides infrastructure and public services to promote e-commerce development and the poor households participate by providing agricultural products and services with the help of agricultural and pastoral cooperatives. Under the operation mode of the "Internet + tourism + special agricultural products," the integrated development of the primary, secondary and tertiary industries is realized, delivering added value and creating more opportunities for the poor households to shake off poverty and get rich in the "Internet +" era.

Source Tang and Lin (2016).

5.3.3 Policies on the Interest Subsidies for Poverty-Relief Loans and the Microloans

In 1986, the People's Bank of China and the Agricultural Bank of China jointly formulated a special policy on the interest subsidies for poverty-relief loans. The credit funds shall be earmarked annually by the People's Bank of China and distributed and managed by the Agricultural Bank of China. The interest subsidies are mostly funded by the central government. The policies on the interest subsidies for poverty-relief loans mainly targeted at the production projects that require small investment, produces quick returns, have a promising market and low entry level for poor households, leverages local resources, and can meet the subsistence needs in short time. The loans shall give priority to small-scale projects in animal farming, aquaculture, agricultural product processing, transport and labor export. The special loans with interest subsidies shall be mainly provided to poor households or joint households for self-use. The poor households could also use the loans to buy shares in the collectives and township enterprises. Various self-financed agricultural, industrial and commercial cooperative economic organizations, township enterprises and a few small county-run industries that provided services or jobs for poor rural households could also apply for the loans. A small number of economic entities with the legal-person status for production, development, operation and services could also, under the premise of voluntary participation, mutual benefit and solvency, serve as a creditor and a debtor for households.

In recent years, the policy on interest subsidy for poverty-relief loans has matured into the policy on microloans for poverty reduction. Since the beginning of registration and accurate identification of poor households in 2014, the policy on microloans has provided the registered poor households with collateral-free small loans, up to RMB 50,000 on a three-year term, at benchmark interest rates, with interest subsidized by government poverty-reduction funds and risk compensation from county-level funds. The microcredit mainly aims to support the registered poor households willing to use loans to develop their businesses and increase income.

References

Han, H., Xu, Y. (2014). Study of anti-poverty effect of China's Rural subsistence allowance system—Empirical Evidence from Five Provinces in Central and Western China. *Economic Review, 6*.

IHA. (2016). Hydropower Status Report 2016, International Hydropower Association.

Kakwani, N., & Pernia, E. M. (2000). What is Pro-poor growth? *Asian Development Review, 18*(1); World Bank. (2016). World development indicators 2016, International Bank for Reconstruction and Development/The World Bank.
Lin, J. Y. (1994). *Institution, technology and agricultural development in China*, Shanghai Sanlian Bookstore, Shanghai People's Publishing House.
Ministry of Civil Affairs. (2016). Statistical Communiqué on Social Service Development 2015.
Ministry of Education, National Development and Reform Commission, and Ministry of Finance. Opinions on Overall Improvement of Basic Conditions of Disadvantaged Schools of Compulsory Education in Poverty-ridden Areas [by Department I of Basic Education, Ministry of Education. (2013) No.10]. Website of Ministry of Education. http://www.moe.gov.cn.
Ministry of Education, National Development and Reform Commission, and Ministry of Finance. Opinions on the Implementation of the 3-year Action Plan for the Second Stage Pre-school Education [by e Department II of Basic Education, Ministry of Education. (2014) No.9]. Website of Ministry of Education: http://www.moe.gov.cn.
National Bureau of Statistics of China. (2016a). The Statistical Communiqué of the People's Republic of China on the 2015 National Economic and Social Development.
National Development and Reform Commission. (2014). National Administrative provisions for work relief. http://www.ndrc.gov.cn.
National Health and Family Planning Commission. (2016b). Interpretations of "Guidelines on the Implementation of the Poverty Reduction Projects through Health Promotion.".
State Council. Opinions of the State Council on Current Development of Preschool Education. (2010). [Guo Fa (2010) No.41]. Website of the central government. http://www.gov.cn.
Tang, Y., Lin, W. (2016). Tibet's exploration in the new path of E-commerce for poverty reduction. *Economic Information Daily*.
The Interpretation of Ministry of Education on the Opinions on Implementing the Second Action Plan for Three-Year Preschool Education. http://www.gov.cn/xinwen/2014-11/16/content2779388.htm.
Wang, X. (2017). *The measurement of poverty: Theories and methods*, Social Sciences Academic Press.

Chapter 6
China's Poverty Reduction Outlook: 2021–2030

To fulfill the goal of building a moderately prosperous society in all respects by 2020, the Chinese government has been engaged in poverty elimination in line with the *Outline for Development-oriented Poverty Reduction for China's Rural Areas (2011–2020)*. The next decade from 2021 to 2030 will be a stage of alleviating relative poverty towards "higher human development." This chapter begins with a brief analysis of the economic and social background of poverty reduction in China between 2021 and 2030, followed by a discussion over the poverty line for the new decade as well as the highlights of the poverty-reduction strategies in pursuit of balanced urban–rural development, before proposing the policy to integrate poverty reduction with sustainable development toward the UN Sustainable Development Goals.

6.1 Background

China has seen steady progress in poverty reduction based on a complete set of strategies. The national poverty-reduction strategies constitute an integral part of China's poverty governance modernization. China has implemented three poverty-reduction strategies by now. The first one is the *Seven-Year Program for Lifting 80 Million People out of Poverty (1994–2000)*, the second one the *Outline for Development-oriented Poverty Reduction for China's Rural Areas (2001–2010)* and the third incorporating the *Outline for Development-oriented Poverty Reduction for China's Rural Areas (2011–2020)*, the *Decision of the CPC Central Committee and the State Council on Eradicating Poverty in China*, and the *National Plan for Poverty Reduction in the 13th Five-Year Plan Period*. National poverty-reduction strategies made strategic arrangements in terms of the actual situation, goals, tasks, subjects, policies, organizations and leadership during a certain period. After the building of a moderately prosperous society in all respects by 2020, the phased characteristics of

X. Wang and X. Zhang, *Towards 2030 – China's Poverty Alleviation and Global Poverty Governance*, International Research on Poverty Reduction,
https://doi.org/10.1007/978-981-15-6356-0_6

China's economic and social development will change accordingly. From the macroeconomic perspective, China will be at a critical stage in the transition from a mid- and high-income country into a high-income country. Judging from the international development, the world will achieve the SDGs by 2030. Under such circumstances, what are the key points for China's poverty-reduction strategy for the upcoming decade and what strategic arrangements should be made to ensure China's fulfilment of the SDGs toward common prosperity? To answer these questions, we first need to conduct a brief analysis of the background for poverty reduction from 2021 to 2030.

6.1.1 Per Capita GDP to Reach USD 10,000

Despite the shift of China's economy from high growth to the new normal of moderately high growth, a range of predictions have affirmed that China's per capita GDP will exceed USD 10,000 in 2020, ranking China among the high-income countries with a per capita GDP of USD 12,000. Justin Lin Yifu said at the 2015 annual meeting of *China Business Times* that China's economy can realize a 6.5% or higher annual growth within the 13th Five-Year Plan period, and that China's per capita GDP may reach USD 12,615 by 2020, potentially making China a high-income country by then.[1] At the China Development Forum 2016 held on March 19, 2016, Wang Yiming, Vice President of the Development Research Center of the State Council, noted that in the 13th Five-Year Plan, the Chinese government has set a target of doubling the 2010 level of GDP and per capita income of urban and rural residents by 2020. In fact, measured against the mid-point exchange rate in 2015, the per capita GDP in 10 of China's 31 provincial-level administrative regions has exceeded USD 10,000, involving a total population of permanent residents of over 500 million. According to the above-mentioned target, China's per capita GDP will reach USD 11,000 by 2020, elevating China from a middle-income country to a high-income one, which means a lot to China and the world. It will require corresponding major adjustments to the poverty-reduction strategies and policies in China. In particular, the criteria for poverty measurement shall be adjusted notably. China's current rural poverty line is RMB 2,300 per person per year (at constant price in 2010). Measured against the 2011 PPP, it equals to USD 2.29 per person per day. The World Bank recommends the consumption-based poverty line of USD 3.1 per person per day for middle-income countries and USD 10 per person per day for high-income countries.

[1] Hui and Lin (2015).

6.1.2 Urban Residents Accounting for Over 60% of the Total Population

According to the national plan, by 2020 the total population will reach about 1.42 billion, with permanent urban residents accounting for 60% and that of urban *hukou*-holding population 45%.[2] It means that the urban population will be much larger than the rural population. Meanwhile, the floating population in China will remain above 200 million. In this context, the government must take the following problems into full consideration in the poverty-reduction strategy for the upcoming decade. First, will China continue with the current separate poverty-reduction strategies and policy systems for rural and urban areas? By now, China's poverty reduction plan, namely the *Outline for Development-oriented Poverty Reduction for China's Rural Areas (2011–2020)*, only targets the rural residents. Despite a series of poverty-alleviating measures, such as subsistence allowance, employment promotion and medical services, there lacks a complete set of poverty-relief strategies for urban China. Second, by 2015 the number of people who live in places other than their household registration area reached 294 million, of which 247 million were floating population.[3] The floating population is estimated to remain above 200 million by 2021. The current structure of the floating population shows that 80% of them move from rural to urban areas. It means that if we continue with the current separate poverty-alleviating strategies for rural and urban China, it would be difficult to identify and help the poor people among the floating population, which is a problem to be solved.

6.1.3 Prominent Aging Problem

China, together with the United States, Brazil, the Russian Federation, and Japan, has the lowest fertility rate in the world, according to UN forecasts.[4] Low fertility and high life expectancy will lead China into a super-aging society by 2030. The Office of China National Committee on Aging predicts that by 2030, 23.3% of the population will be aged 60 or above (see Fig. 6.1). Some experts think that China's latest two-child policy will slow down the aging trend, but the trend is irreversible, posing a challenge for China's poverty reduction from 2021 to 2030.

Along with urbanization and population movements came a growing body of "empty nests" and "left-behind" seniors in rural China, particularly in poverty-stricken rural areas where an increasing number of the elderly lost the ability to

---

[2]Report on the Work of the Government delivered at the Fourth Session of the 12th National People's Congress of the People's Republic of China by Premier Li Keqiang on March 5, 2016.

[3]National Bureau of Statistics of China. Statistical Communiqué of the People's Republic of China on the 2015 National Economic and Social Development. March 1, 2016.

[4]United Nations Department of Economic and Social Affairs/Population Division. World Population Prospects: The 2015 Revision, Key Findings and Advance Tables. United Nations, New York, 2015.

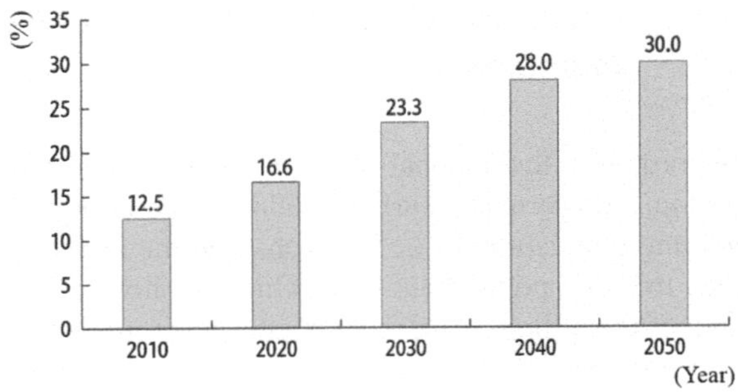

Fig. 6.1 Ratio of people over 60 in China. *Source* Yushao Wu. *China Report of the Development on Old-Age Services (2013)*. Social Sciences Academic Press (China). 2013

work because of aging, illness or disability. This has posed the most severe challenge to the strategy and policies of development-oriented poverty reduction since its launch in 1986. Therefore, it has become a must for China to reform the poverty-alleviating models and explore new strategies and policies befitting the new stage of aging and urbanization.

6.1.4 Rising Dependency Ratio as a Result of the "Two-Child Policy"

In 2015, China proposed to implement the policy of allowing two children for every couple ("two-child policy" in short) in an active response to the aging problem. However, the children born under the new policy won't reach working age until after 2030. In other words, the "two-child policy" will not help expand the labor force before 2030. On the other hand, the policy will translate into a notably higher dependency ratio by changing the family structure from "4-2-1" (four elders—a couple—a child) to "4-2-2."[5] The expenditures on education, healthcare and others will increase accordingly.

6.1.5 Ecological Challenges for Poverty Reduction

In response to the UN's 2030 SDGs, the Chinese government has put forward the vision of green development.[6] Green development, representing an eco-friendly

[5]The "4-2-1" family structure means that under the previous "one-child policy", each couple has to support four elders and raise one child. The "4-2-2" family structure means that under the new "two child policy", each couple will have to support four elders and raise two children.

[6]According to the CPC Central Committee Recommendations for the 13th Five-Year Plan for Economic and Social Development passed on October 29, 2015, to achieve the development goals for the 13th Five-Year Plan period, resolve major difficulties in development and cultivate strengths to be applied to development, it's a must to promote innovative, coordinated, green, open, and

outlook, is both a necessary condition to sustain development and a manifestation of the people's pursuit for a better life. We must implement the fundamental national policy of conserving resources and protecting the environment, pursue a model of sustainable development featuring increased production, higher living standards, and healthy ecosystems, step up efforts to build a resource-conserving and environmentally-friendly society, promote modernization featuring harmonious development between Man and Nature, and continue the "Beautiful China" initiative to play our part in ensuring global ecological security.[7]

The distribution of poverty-stricken counties highly overlaps with that of national eco-function zones. The key eco-function zones identified in the *National Plan for Developing Functional Zones* [Guo Fa (2010) No.46] cover 436 county-level administrative regions, of which 310 are poverty-stricken. These counties undertake key ecological functions such as national water resource conservation, soil conservation, wind prevention and sand fixation, and biodiversity conservation. Industrial development is generally forbidden in these areas. In the meanwhile, most poor counties suffer from fragile ecological environment and frequent natural disasters. To help the poor population in these areas, it's necessary to explore ways to achieve human development, in particular poverty eradication, in a sustainable way while formulating the poverty-alleviating strategies for the period from 2021 to 2030.

6.2 New Poverty Line: 2030 and Beyond

The poverty line is vital for formulating poverty reduction strategies and policies, identifying the poor population and providing targeted assistance. What poverty line does China need for poverty reduction between 2021 and 2030? Let's start with a brief international comparative analysis.

6.2.1 Basic Approaches to Defining the Poverty Line

So far there are three basic approaches to define the poverty line in the world: the basic needs approach, income threshold approach and basic capabilities approach, corresponding to three measurements of "absolute poverty," "relative poverty" and "multidimensional poverty."

shared development, also known as the "Five Development Concepts". As we can see that green development is one of the five concepts.

[7]The CPC Central Committee Recommendations for the 13th Five-Year Plan for Economic and Social Development passed on October 29, 2015.

1. The basic needs approach

The basic needs approach defines income- or consumption-based poverty line in terms of the amount of money required to fulfill the basic needs for survival, including the basic needs for food and non-food items, such as clothing and sheltering. In his book *Poverty: A Study of Town Life* published in 1901, British scholar Benjamin Seebohm Rowntree estimated the poverty line in the city of York, England by estimating the budget required for the "shopping basket" to "obtain the minimum necessities for the maintenance of merely physical efficiency." Rowntree concluded that 15 shillings would provide the minimum budget for food for a family of six for one week. Adding an allowance for shelter, clothing, fuel and sundries, he arrived at a poverty line of 26 shillings for a family of six for one week that implied a poverty rate of almost 10% in York at the time. This is the earliest practice of defining poverty in terms of the amount of money required to satisfy the basic needs for food and non-food items. Prior to 1950, the UK used the "shopping basket" to meet the basic needs for food, clothing and sheltering to measure the poverty level. The approach was later adopted by the USA and most countries and has been in use ever since. It is also used by the World Bank to define the international poverty line.

Following this approach, the absolute poverty line is determined based on the basic needs for food and non-food items. It first estimates the cost of acquiring enough rice (flour), vegetable, meat (milk, egg) at market prices for adequate nutrition—usually 2,100 or 2,300 calories per person per day. Then, based on the proportion of the non-food consumption to the overall household consumption, it estimates the cost for non-food essentials. The two costs would add up to the absolute poverty line. In the low-income countries, the food expenditure usually accounts for 60% of the total household expenditure (Engel's coefficient) and the non-food expenditure 40%. The poverty line in the USA is determined based on a proportion of 1/3 for food expenditure and 2/3 for non-food expenditure.

Generally speaking, along with the economic and social development, the publicly acceptable basic needs would increase correspondingly, so does the poverty line. Among developed countries, the USA was the first to establish its absolute poverty line according to the basic needs approach in 1963, which is still in use today. Developed countries generally set different poverty lines for different family structures and sizes. In 2015, the poverty line for a family of four (a couple with two children) in the USA was USD 24,000, about USD 16.50 per person per day (see Table 6.1). In 2015, the poor population in the USA was 43.1 million, making up 13.5% of the total population.

So far, the basic needs approach has been adopted by more than 80 developing countries in the world to set the absolute poverty line, but the general pattern is that the higher the per capita GDP, the higher the absolute poverty line.

2. The relative income approach

The relative income approach defines relative poverty based on a certain proportion of the median income. This approach is more commonly used in the EU and the UK.

Table 6.1 The US poverty line for 2015, (USD per year)

Size of family	Weighted average poverty thresholds	Minors under 18								
		0	1	2	3	4	5	6	7	8 or more
One person (unrelated individual)	12,082									
Under 65	12,331	12,331								
65 and over	11,367	11,367								
Two people	15,391									
Householder under 65	15,952	15,871	16,337							
Householder aged 65 and over	14,342	14,326	16,275							
Three people	18,871	18,540	19,078	19,096						
Four people	24,257	24,447	24,847	24,036	24,120					
Five people	28,741	29,482	29,911	28,995	28,286	27,853				
Six people	32,542	33,909	34,044	33,342	32,670	31,670	31,078			
Seven people	36,998	39,017	39,260	38,421	37,835	36,745	35,473	34,077		
Eight people	41,029	43,637	44,023	43,230	42,536	41,551	40,300	38,999	38,668	
Nine people or more.	49,177	52,493	52,747	52,046	51,457	50,490	49,159	47,956	47,658	45,822

Source U.S. Census Bureau. September 2016

Table 6.2 Cash value of poverty lines for different family types in 2013–2014, (£ per week)

Family types	Relative poverty line
Single adult	134
Childless couple	232
Couple, 1 child	278
Lone parent,1 child	181
Couple, 3 children	371

Source Living Standards, Poverty and Inequality in the UK: 2015. The Institute for Fiscal Studies
Note The data for income refers to the income after housing cost

In 1979, the UK defined the relative poverty line as the 60% of median household income. Median income refers to the after-tax income earned by households in the middle of income distribution. The UK government calculated the cash value of poverty lines for different types of families with less than 60% of the median income (see Table 6.2). The UK government also applied the approach to set the absolute poverty line, defining the population with "household income below 60% of the median income in 2010" as absolutely poor. In 2014, the relative poverty line for a couple with one child in the UK was £278 a week, about £13.2 per person per day. In 2014, the relatively poor population accounted for 21% of the total in the UK. Since it's difficult to evaluate the government's performance in poverty reduction in terms of the relative poverty standard, the EU countries tended to return to the absolute poverty line in recent years.

Both the UK and the USA establish different poverty standards, whether it be relative or absolute, for different types of families. It's conducive to attributing targeted social welfare to different family types while preventing "splitting households" for the benefit of social welfare.

3. The basic capabilities approach

In recent years, with the advancement of human society, a large number of low-income countries have climbed up to the ranks of middle-income countries and more attention is given to the access to basic capabilities, such as education, health services and employment. The commonly held view is that increasing income is only a means to promote development-oriented poverty reduction, but the improvement of capabilities, or human development, should be the ultimate purpose. For instance, the per capita income of RMB 2,300 in rural China is only a means to shake off poverty; the ultimate goal is "two no-worries and three guarantees."[8] In this context, the new poverty standard measured by multidimensional poverty index is extended widely in the world. As of today, over 40 countries have established

[8]"Two no-worries and three guarantees" is the ultimate goal stated in the *Outline for Development-oriented Poverty Reduction for China's Rural Areas (2011–2020)*, ensuring that the impoverished rural population no longer has to worry about food and clothing, with guaranteed compulsory education, basic medical treatment and housing security.

their own multidimensional poverty standard. In particular, Latin American countries, such as Brazil, Colombia and Mexico, have formulated poverty standards from multiple dimensions like education, health, youth development and employment to narrow the development gap. The UNDP also adopted the multidimensional poverty index in 2010.

In the practice of development-oriented poverty reduction in China, the above three approaches have co-existed. The national rural poverty line is in fact based on the basic needs approach. In recent years, Zhejiang Province has established relative poverty standards by means of the relative income approach. According to the *Opinions on Establishing a Poverty Delisting Mechanism*, the poor families can be removed from the poverty record if they have a stable annual per capita net income above the national poverty line, with guaranteed access to food, clothing, compulsory education, basic health insurance and housing security. This is actually a multidimensional poverty standard combining "basic needs" with "basic capabilities."

6.2.2 China's Poverty Policy Options for 2030

1. China needs to introduce multidimensional poverty criteria

Pin–kun is a combination of *pin*, meaning lack of income, and *kun* (hardships), limited access to services such as education, health, housing, social security and employment. The State Council Leading Group of Poverty Alleviation and Development, the government body for poverty reduction, comprises representatives from over 40 departments that each plays an important role in the country's poverty-reduction campaigns. Apart from providing assistance or increasing the poor's income, the leading group is also committed to helping them overcome such difficulties in access to water, electricity, roads and other basic facilities and limited access to public services including education, health and social security. China's poverty-reduction policies are not only about income generation through business promotion, job creation or other means; they are also designed to ensure better access to infrastructure and public services. They are thus multidimensional, aiming at improving economic, social, environmental and other aspects of life. Therefore, we propose a multidimensional poverty line be developed for the period from 2021 to 2030. This would be in consistence with the multiple criteria used before 2020 to evaluate whether a household is lifted out of poverty.[9]

---

[9]By 2020, the criteria to evaluate whether a household could be lifted out of poverty incorporates an annual per capita net income that keeps the household above the national poverty threshold, adequate food and clothing, guaranteed access to compulsory education and basic healthcare, and a secure place to live.

2. The basic framework of the multidimensional poverty standard

China's multidimensional poverty standard is suitable for the stage of economic and social development and consistent with the targeted poverty-reduction strategy and the development-oriented poverty-reduction concept. It's a comprehensive standard to evaluate the "lack" of income and "hardships" in the fields other than income, incorporating income-based poverty and non-income poverty. According to the Opinions on Establishing a Poverty Delisting Mechanism, the standard for poverty delisting combines the income-based poverty standard with the guaranteed access to food, clothing, compulsory education, basic health insurance and housing security. This is a multidimensional poverty standard that takes both "lack" and "hardships" into consideration, pointing the way for poverty standard formulation and poverty identification during the decade from 2021 to 2030.

The income-based poverty standard could be further raised in line with the development stage to align it with the per capita GDP. The "basic needs approach" should be applied to determine the list of food for basic needs and the proportion of non-food essentials, in a bid to calculate the absolute poverty line in terms of income or consumption.

As for the non-income poverty standard, the poverty dimensions should be further expanded on the basis of the current standard of "the guaranteed access to food, clothing, compulsory education, basic health insurance and housing security," while raising the standard for each dimension and indicator. Such dimensions may involve education, health, housing, living standards and employment. For example, in the dimension of education, the nine-year compulsory education could be extended to 12 or 15 years. In the dimension of health, the indicators for safe drinking water, sanitary latrines, clean household energy and others could be further improved.

Furthermore, given that the 2021–2030 period will be crucial for China's urbanization, the poverty of over 200 million floating people will present new characteristics. The social inclusion of the new immigrants to cities, especially those from the rural areas, should be a major concern. Having got rid of material poverty, they are still in relative poverty in terms of cultural or subjective welfare. Drawing on lessons from the problems facing the middle-income countries in Latin America, we believe that it's necessary to regard social inclusion as a dimension for future poverty standard or poverty-related measurement and evaluation. The framework of China's multidimensional poverty standard from 2021 to 2030 is shown in Table 6.3.

The weights of income poverty and non-income poverty, income-based poverty standards, as well as the dimensions, indicators and weights of non-income poverty should be studied and formulated jointly by the State Council Leading Group for Poverty Alleviation and Development, the National Bureau of Statistics and other relevant government bodies.

Table 6.3 Framework of China's multidimensional poverty standard from 2021 to 2030

Classification	Dimension	Description
Lack (in income/consumption)	Per capita income/consumption	Could meet the basic food and non-food needs acceptable to the Chinese society between 2021 and 2030 to guarantee human dignity
Hardships (non-income)	Education	15-year compulsory education Early childhood education for the 0–3-year-olds Preschool education for the 4–6-year-olds
	Health	Basic medical insurance for all Serious disease insurance subsidies for the poor Serious disease assistance for the poor
	Housing	Security Per capita area above a certain criterion
	Living standards	Safe drinking water Sanitary toilet Clean cooking fuel Possession of the washing machine, refrigerator and Mobile phone
	Employment	Jobs for capable working-age people Capable working-age people master at least one skill
	Social inclusion in cities	Sense of belonging in cities and communities (threshold could be set based on the subject's personal feelings)

3. Adjustment of multidimensional poverty standards

The comprehensive poverty index, including dimensions and indicators, are adjusted every five years along with the five-year plan for national economic and social development, by expanding the range of dimensions and indicators and raising the poverty threshold of each indicator.

To sum up, the comprehensive poverty index serves the purpose of poverty assessment standard befitting Chinese definition of poverty, administration of poverty reduction in China, development-oriented poverty-reduction policy system, and the targeted poverty-reduction strategy. It's an integral part of the development-oriented poverty reduction with Chinese characteristics. Based on the comprehensive poverty index, the National Bureau of Statistics calculates the national poor population and the incidence of poverty, the State Council Leading Group Office of Poverty Alleviation and Development devises the methods for poverty identification, the local governments set the indicators and scores for poverty identification, and other related departments provide targeted assistance to the poor people accordingly.

6.3 Coordinating Poverty Reduction in Urban and Rural Areas

6.3.1 Poverty Monitoring for Both Urban and Rural Residents

The existing national poverty monitoring system mainly targets at rural poverty. With the reform of the household registration system and the advancement of urbanization, it is necessary to establish a poverty monitoring system covering both urban and rural residents. China has unified the survey for urban and rural households and is now conducting the survey of income, expenditure and living conditions of households nationwide, which laid the foundation for poverty monitoring for both urban and rural residents. The development-oriented poverty-reduction system and subsistence allowance system in rural China are two pillars for the battle against poverty. The subsistence allowance system is extended from urban to rural areas. The next step is to extend the development-oriented poverty-reduction system from rural to urban areas on the basis of coordinated urban–rural poverty monitoring.

6.3.2 Unified Poverty Standards for Both Urban and Rural Residents

Poverty is not peculiar to rural residents; it is a serious problem facing urban residents as well. When China began to establish poverty reduction institutions and advance the development-oriented poverty reduction in an organized and large-scale manner in 1986, it was primarily an agricultural country, so it made sense to focus its anti-poverty institutions on rural China. But in the upcoming decade from 2021 to 2030, the ratio of urban residents to the national population in China will far exceed that of rural residents. Judging from the poverty situation in middle-income countries, urban poverty will emerge as the main form of poverty with the advancement of urbanization. Moreover, the consequences of urban poverty may be more difficult to manage than those of rural poverty. It's necessary to establish a unified urban–rural poverty standard to accurately understand the country's poverty situation, so as to formulate corresponding poverty-reduction strategies and policies.

6.3.3 Coordinated Urban–Rural Poverty-Reduction Strategies

In the future, "development-oriented poverty reduction" and "subsistence allowances" would continue to constitute the main framework of China's poverty-reduction system. But development-oriented poverty-reduction programs should be extended to include urban residents.

For programs targeting urban residents, employment should be at the core. A coordinated urban–rural poverty-reduction strategy requires long-term strategic planning for the development of human capital through education, health and so on, while making "investment in people, in children and in the future" a long-term institutional arrangement for poverty reduction in the new stage. In addition, the urban–rural development-oriented poverty-reduction strategy should align with the "Made in China 2025" and the Belt and Road Initiative to transform and upgrade the labor force. Institutional arrangements must be made to address the new challenges posed by the "aging society" and "two-child policy."

Regarding the poverty-reduction policies for the decade from 2021 to 2030, we may consider supporting the development of such emerging industries as elderly care, leisure, child services and environmental protection to supplement the decades-long role of industrial development in poverty reduction.

6.4 Poverty Reduction and Sustainable Development

Green development is one of the "Five Development Concepts" being implemented in China, proposed in response to a series of severe environmental problems such as the pollution of air, water and land, which are growing ever more prominently. The UN SDGs 2030 integrate poverty governance with sustainable development as well. Therefore, both domestic situation and the common goal of the international community require China to integrate poverty reduction with sustainable development in the 2021–2030 decade.

6.4.1 Establish an Institutional Framework Featuring Close Integration of Poverty Reduction with Sustainable Development

The *National Plan for Poverty Reduction in the 13th Five-Year Plan Period* dedicated a chapter to "poverty reduction through ecological conservation," elevating it to a standalone policy for development-oriented poverty reduction since the launch of the large-scale development-oriented poverty reduction in 1986, and marking an outstanding progress in theory and practice of China's development-oriented poverty reduction. We're confident that the five-year anti-poverty fight will give rise to a number of good practices and valuable experience in all localities, which will be a great boon for the development-oriented poverty reduction after 2020.

Following the five-year exploration of poverty reduction through ecological conservation from 2016 to 2000, the next step is to embed the concept of sustainable development into each poverty reduction policy. For example, the work relief programs, relocation programs, industrial development and all other programs or policies for development-oriented poverty reduction should be designed to pursue sustainable and green development. It will increase the cost of development-oriented poverty reduction, but it's worthwhile in the long run.

6.4.2 Establish the PPES Mechanism

The mechanism of Pro-poor Payments for Environmental Services (PPES) is based on the existing Payments for Environmental Services (PES) mechanism, with the purpose of maximizing the benefits for the poor people through ecological transfer payments. China has implemented for years the Grain for Green Program and the policies to subsidize people who protect the grassland ecology, generating transfer income for the poor. With the rising ecological value and its external benefits, we need to increase the subsidies for ecological services and the compensation for the poor.

As the fiscal transfer payment from the government is limited, it is necessary to open up the ecological compensation market and explore the mechanism for enterprises, social organizations and even individual citizens to purchase ecological services. In this context, it's necessary to open up the carbon trading market, particularly to develop more convenient tools for carbon calculating and trading tools. The unprecedented development of remote sensing, GIS and big data technology has provided strong technical support for a more convenient carbon trading environment.

6.4.3 Promote Carbon Financing Innovation and "Low-Carbon Poverty Reduction"[10]

1. Set up a steering group for "low-carbon poverty reduction" to promote carbon financing in poor areas. To help poverty-stricken areas and people participate in carbon financing, the priority is to remove technical barriers. To this end, it's advisable to set up a steering group composed of government bodies, research institutes, enterprises and local farmers in poverty-stricken areas. The group shall be responsible for: (1) in line with the characteristics of local poverty reduction work, studying how to build a financial platform for "low-carbon poverty

[10] Ji and Wang (2012).

reduction," incorporating government finance, carbon trading market, carbon fund, green credit, and so on, and establishing a domestic inter-regional carbon financing mechanism under the existing framework of "collaboration on poverty reduction between the eastern and western regions"; (2) setting the course for the future development of the poor areas, exploring the agricultural projects with development potential and seeking international partners; (3) making technical preparations for project application; (4) categorizing the projects and standardizing the operation model and approval procedures for each category; (5) drawing up experience and lessons and formulating a guide for "low-carbon poverty reduction" covering technical specifications, operational procedures, policy framework and others; (6) assessing the project's pro-poor effects and continuously improving the carbon financing framework in the poor areas; (7) developing pilot programs of "low-carbon poverty reduction"; (8) organizing awareness-raising and training programs to promote sharing and exchange.

2. Develop agricultural CDM projects to further promote development-oriented poverty reduction. We should help poor rural areas seize opportunities and develop locally appropriate agricultural and forestry CDM projects, in order to generate additional income for local farmers and foster local industry with competitive edge.
3. Develop voluntary programs for emission reduction, promote voluntary carbon trading market and encourage multi-stakeholder participation in "low-carbon poverty reduction." In response to the requirements of "social responsibility" and "carbon neutrality," we will develop voluntary programs for emission reduction, promote voluntary trading markets, and encourage enterprises, individuals and other sectors of the society to participate in "low-carbon poverty reduction." We will advance the development of market for voluntary emission reduction in China. With a view for the development of agricultural CDM projects, we will put in place the certification, pricing and registration systems for voluntary emission reduction programs which are consistent with national conditions and compatible with international regulations, and once they are mature, align them with the corresponding overseas registration and trading systems, in an effort to promote them internationally. In the meanwhile, we need to step up the publicity work. With the help of brochures and media, we will publicize the means of low-carbon poverty reduction through voluntary emission reduction among enterprise, communities and individuals. We will set up charity financing channels for low-carbon poverty reduction and channel the carbon funds in the voluntary market for emission reduction to poverty-reduction programs.
4. Set up a special fund for "low-carbon poverty reduction," encourage the participation of financial institutions and establish a "unilateral model for low-carbon poverty reduction." The special fund shall support agricultural and forestry projects that cannot be registered under the bilateral model. The CERs obtained by these projects could be purchased with the special fund. The CERs account or stock could be set up to facilitate the trading with other institutions in carbon market. The yields thus generated could be used to supplement the special fund

or distributed to the participating farmers in the form of work relief.By encouraging the participation of banks, we can further promote the financing for the "unilateral model" of low-carbon poverty reduction. The deep involvement of Indian banking institutions has contributed to the prosperity of the unilateral model of emission reduction in the country, which is enlightening for China. The agricultural and forestry projects in poverty-stricken areas are entitled to preferential loans from banks. The CERs obtained can be stored in financial institutions or traded in the market by project developers for the repayment of loans. The existing Equator Principles serve as an important guidance for commercial banks to fulfill their social responsibilities, but by now, they only have one signatory in China: the Industrial Bank. It is recommended to urge other commercial banks to issue "low-carbon poverty reduction credits," in a bid to play an active part in the investment and financing for low-carbon poverty reduction while fulfilling their social responsibilities.

5. Make active effort to apply for international carbon funds and develop the "multilateral model for low-carbon poverty reduction." Enterprises should be mobilized to provide financial aid for the establishment of a low-carbon poverty-reduction fund, so as to help poor areas actively apply for international multilateral carbon funds. In particular, for the projects that have difficulty in finding buyers, great efforts should be made to seek for the assistance from international carbon funds, such as the World Bank BioCarbon Fund and the Forest Carbon Partnership Facility Fund—both are open to applicants from developing countries.
6. Help poor areas to develop PCDM (Programmatic CDM) projects and increase the scale and efficiency of carbon financing in these areas. PCDM is to integrate the emission-reduction measures relating to a specific sustainable development policy into an overall plan to register, certify and issue corresponding CERs as a whole. On the basis of international and domestic experience, we will help poor areas integrate different projects according to various rules through the PCDM framework, especially for household biogas, solar energy, energy-efficient lamp projects which are dispersive, popular and consumable and produce less emission. Such integrations could be conducted by technology, by greenhouse gas or by industry, start at a micro level and gradually extend to a larger scale. In the meanwhile, the operation mode and approval procedures for each category of integrated projects shall be standardized, so as to improve the project efficiency and facilitate their promotion on a large scale.

References

Hui, J., & Lin, J. L. (2015). China's per capita GDP may reach USD 12,615 by 2020. *Economic Information Daily*.

Ji, X., & Wang, X. (2012). Carbon financing innovation and "low-carbon poverty reduction." *Issues in Agricultural Economy, 1*.

Chapter 7
Reflections on the Current State of Global Poverty Governance

From the perspective of global poverty governance, this chapter analyzes the evolution of the global poverty governance concepts since the World War II and the status quo and adjustment of international poverty governance since the new millennium.

7.1 An Overview of Global Poverty Governance

The world poverty map indicates that Africa, South Asia, Latin America and Small Island States are in poverty, while the sub-Saharan African countries are in extreme poverty and thus the key focus of global poverty governance. These areas are typically characterized by a large poor population, low productivity, and poor education and medical conditions. Diverse groups of actors are offering assistance to them in different ways to ease these bottlenecks to development.

7.1.1 International Poverty Reduction Agencies

In general, the main forces currently engaged in global poverty governance fall into the following three categories.

1. The mainstay of bilateral assistances

The poverty reduction cooperation among nations mainly takes the form of bilateral assistance which is mainly provided by the member countries of the Organization for Economic Co-operation and Development's Development Assistance Committee (OECD-DAC). Against the backdrop of sluggish global economy ever since the 2008 global financial crisis, the official development assistance (ODA) from the DAC

X. Wang and X. Zhang, *Towards 2030 – China's Poverty Alleviation and Global Poverty Governance*, International Research on Poverty Reduction,
https://doi.org/10.1007/978-981-15-6356-0_7

countries has been diminishing along with their enthusiasm for such assistance. In stark contrast, non-DAC countries have been increasingly active in international bilateral assistance in recent years. In particular, there has been a hefty increase in the volume, scope and fields of assistance provided by emerging countries represented by BRICS countries.

2. Multilateral assistance agencies

Multilateral development assistance organizations fall into three broad categories: international multilateral banks, international multilateral financial organizations and international multilateral development institutions. Among the multilateral banks, the World Bank has played the most active role in global poverty reduction, followed by regional banks such as the Asian Development Bank, the African Development Bank and the Asian Infrastructure Investment Bank. The multilateral financial organizations include the International Monetary Fund—the most active among them, and the International Fund for Agricultural Development (IFAD). The international multilateral development agencies mainly refer to agencies under the United Nations which is an international organization of sovereign states founded after the World War II. For example, the UN Economic and Social Council is the main agency responsible for global poverty governance; the United Nations Food and Agriculture Organization (FAO), United Nations Educational, Scientific and Cultural Organization (UNESCO), United Nations Development Programme (UNDP), and United Nations Children's Fund (UNICEF) have each established special organs for poverty reduction and governance.

3. A wide array of international NGOs, foundations, charities, individuals, etc.

Huge in number but scattered around the world, they serve as the "capillaries" of global poverty governance, including the Bill & Melinda Gates Foundation, the Ford Foundation and the Oxfam. Deeply rooted in communities and boasting wide public support, they enthusiastically mobilize the community residents and volunteers to engage in poverty-reduction programs. After the financial crisis, developed countries have introduced reforms to traditional bilateral assistance, and introduced the public–private partnership (PPP) for to increase support for domestic NGOs and social enterprises while launching overseas aid programs.

7.1.2 Evolution of Global Poverty Governance

Not all international development agencies have made poverty reduction their main task since the very beginning, and not all ODAs are designed to serve the poor people.

It's widely believed that US's Marshall Plan in the Europe and the "Point Four Program" (a technical assistance program for backward regions) in developing countries heralded the beginning for the international development assistance to play its role around the world. To sum up, with the collapse of the Soviet Union in the 1990s as the main watershed, the evolution of international development assistance can be divided into two stages: the pre-Cold War stage and the post-Cold War stage.

1. Establishment of international development assistance

Following the end of the World War II in 1945, countries were faced with the severe challenge of post-war reconstruction: the economy and public infrastructure were paralyzed, and economic development became the priority. To rebuild the world order, bilateral and multilateral organizations and international aid agencies sprouted and began to participate in the economic development of various countries, represented by the establishment of the UN and the World Bank. The US' Marshall Plan and "Point Four Program" marked the beginning of bilateral organizations' participation in the post-war economic recovery of various countries. International NGOs, such as Oxfam and Care International, were set up afterwards. These actions and frameworks showed that the international development assistance system was taking shape.

From the launch of Marshall Plan in 1948 to the 1960s, norms were gradually developed for international development assistance. In particular, international organizations represented by the UN and the OECD pushed forward the developed countries' planned and organized assistance to the economically backward countries. In addition, a growing number of such assistance programs led to the increase in the volume of international development assistance. The 1960s and 1970s were dubbed as the Golden Age of international assistance, but the assistance in this period was obviously political. With the onset of a debt crisis in the developing world during the early 1980s, the US initiated the "Washington Consensus" to promote reforms in market and private economy in developing countries. Such economic reforms later evolved into political intervention that contributed to the ever-widening gap between developed countries and developing ones.

2. Adjustment and redevelopment of international development assistance

The 1990s marked the lowest point for international development assistance which was shrinking in volume for the whole decade. Between 1990 and 1996, the volume of international development assistance dropped by about 20%.[1] The main cause was that such assistance became less important politically for developed countries after the collapse of the socialist camp. As a result, global poverty was worsened from 1991 to 2000. It is not until the adoption of *UN Millennium Declaration* and the Millennium Development Goals in 2000 did the international development assistance enter a new stage after the end of the Cold War.

Prior to the Cold War, the international assistance was active but not ideal in effect. Apart from the Republic of Korea and Taiwan of China, the rest developing world saw little progress in development and some regions even slipped back. Facing the development challenge such as the famine in Africa and debt crisis in Latin America, the international community had to adjust the international development assistance.

[1] Li et al. (2009).

3. Poverty reduction as an important part of international development assistance

Despite its contribution to economic development and poverty alleviation, the international aid prior to the Cold War was too political to produce the desired effect. In 1969, the *Pearson Commission (Report)* published by the World Bank reviewed and reflected on the UN's decade-long international development assistance. While affirming its achievements, the report noted that the assistance paid excessive attention to overall economic growth while ignoring the income distribution and assistance to the poor. It called for more attention and assistance to the poor people. In particular, the foreign aid of developed countries should be raised to 0.7% of the GNP. In the 1970s, the World Bank and the United Nations launched the Integrated Rural Development Project (IRDP) to provide multilateral assistance for poverty reduction in rural areas of developing countries. Subsequently, more similar projects with clear goals in poverty reduction are organized and implemented by countries engaged in bilateral aids.

7.1.3 Development Trend of Global Poverty Governance

1. From results-oriented to process-oriented development

The United Nations issued Millennium Development Goals (MDGs) in 2000 and Sustainable Development Goals (SDGs) in 2015. The changes from MDGs to SDGs actually reflected the shift in the focus of international development assistance from results to process.

As the name suggests, the SDGs emphasize sustainability in the course of development. The goal should be to help the poor acquire more capabilities and rights in the process of development, instead of simply pursuing for growth in GDP and reduction in poor population. As to development goals, the MDGs have eight clearly-defined targets that are easy to market and remember. According to Markus Loewe, the MDGs are SMART goals: Specific, Measurable, Agreed upon, Realistic and Time-bound.[2] However, it's obvious that the MDGs only take the development results into account, while ignoring the impact of the development process and programs. For instance, the poverty-reduction goal among the MDGs stresses the target for the poor population and extreme poverty, while ignoring the well-being and living environment of the disadvantaged people. In terms of the executive body, as introduced in the first chapter, MDGs excessively emphasize the role of aids from developed countries, but ignored the initiative of the recipient countries.

---

[2]Loewe (2014).

2. From North-to-South assistance to South–South cooperation

Following the end of the World War II, a vast number of developing countries successively got rid of colonial rule and set about domestic reconstruction. Following the Bandung Conference in 1955, a large body of the third world countries embarked on a development path of solidarity and close cooperation. Similar to the North-to-South assistance, South–South cooperation was highly political at the beginning, initiated as the antithesis of North-South assistance: North-to-South assistance advocates "conditional aid and political reform," upholds the "Washington Consensus," and has clearly defined recipients and boundaries while South–South cooperation upholds "non-interference in internal affairs, equality, independence, and autonomy" and pursues "economic and trade cooperation for mutual benefits" and "cooperation in diversified fields and forms."

If we say that the main promoter of North-to-South assistance is OECD-DAC, the main driver of South–South cooperation is the United Nations which endorsed the establishment of the Special Unit of South-South Cooperation (SUSSC) in 1974 and the Special Unit for Technical Cooperation among Developing Countries (TCDC) in 2004. In the meanwhile, it also helped found a host of international alliances of developing countries, such as the "Group of 77."

3. From competition to collaboration and integration

The 1980s witnessed a downturn in the North-to-South assistance and the South–South cooperation. After the launch of MDGs after the Cold War, both embraced a new stage of development. However, as the implementation of MDGs took a battering due to the financial crisis, the performance of traditional developed countries was barely satisfactory, while the emerging economies represented by the BRICS countries made eye-catching progress. The lessons from the financial crisis reminded the world that against the backdrop of globalization, the world has entered a stage of nested development. In this context, the North-to-South assistance and South–South cooperation won't thrive separately. Based on such understanding, developed and developing countries have conducted effective cooperation. For instance, the G8 began to invite developing countries to participate as observers in discussions and developed countries are invited to contribute to initiatives of developing countries, such as the Asian Infrastructure Investment Bank.

7.2 Representative International Multilateral Organizations and Their Poverty-Reduction Strategies

7.2.1 HIPC Program

Globally, in addition to the afore-mentioned MDGs and SDGs of the UN, there are Heavily Indebted Poor Countries (HIPC) program and Poverty Reduction and Growth Facility (PRGF) established by the World Bank and the IMF since the 1990s.

In Africa, many countries are in perennial debt and have fallen into the "debt trap" featuring a cycle of borrowing—becoming indebted—re-borrowing—paying debt with loans. Among the creditors are sovereign countries and development financing institutions such as the World Bank and the IMF. To ease the debt burdens of developing countries, especially those in Africa, the World Bank and the IMF launched the HIPC program. By virtue of the joint efforts of the international financial organizations, creditors and debtors, the HIPC program aims to reduce the debt of qualifying HIPC, but the waived debts must be used for national poverty reduction. The program also aims to assist those countries overwhelmed by the debts to formulate new development strategies and steer the least developed countries onto a path of sustainable development. In 1999, the World Bank and the IMF completed a comprehensive review of the program, refined and improved the loan mechanism, and officially initiated the HPIC program. In 2005, in response to the UN MDGs, the World Bank and the African Development Fund (ADF) finalized the Multilateral Debt Relief Initiative (MDRI) that provided 100% debt relief for eligible HIPCs. As of 2014, 36 countries had received the full amount of debt relief.

The HIPC program is a two-stage initiative: the decision-making stage and the completion stage. In the decision-making stage, or to say the preparation stage, the applying country must meet the following four conditions. First, the country is eligible for the interest-free loans and grants provided by the World Bank and the IMF, in other words, identified as poor by the two organizations. Second, the country faces an unsustainable debt burden that cannot be addressed through traditional debt-relief mechanisms and carries out reforms with the help of the World Bank or the IMF. Third, the country has established a track record of reform and sound policies with the help of the IMF and the World Bank. Fourth, the country has developed a nationwide Poverty Reduction Strategy Paper (PRSP). Once the country's eligibility for these four criteria is affirmed by the HIPC Executive Boards and the World Bank, it can move on to the second stage: the completion stage. In this stage, the country must meet the following three criteria. First, it must establish a traceable evaluation system with the help of the IMF and the World Bank. Second, it must implement key reforms agreed. Third, it must adopt and implement its PRSP for at least one year. That is to say, the completion stage of the debt-relief application is actually the beginning stage of the PRSP.

From the macroeconomic perspective, the HIPC program has improved the finances of the poor countries effectively and given a break to the least developed countries overwhelmed by debts. But we notice the influence of the PRSP developed by the IMF and the World Bank in the implementation process, whose effect is worth re-examination for the PRSP is not a national poverty-reduction strategy befitting the national conditions, but a "development plan" forced upon the country based on the poverty-reduction concepts of developed countries.

7.2.2 Poverty Reduction and Growth Trust

In 1999, the IMF established the Poverty Reduction and Growth Facility (PRGF) to benefit its poorest member countries. In 2002 and 2004, the PRGF project team and Independent Evaluation Office (IEO) of the IMF evaluated the project and proposed reforms to adapt to the increasing public expenditures.[3] In the report *The IMF and Aid to Sub-Saharan Africa* issued by IEO in 2007, IEO recommended that to sustain the economic growth and put the loans into effective use, it's necessary to integrate the PRGF program with international development assistance and enhance the management of international assistance to make the funds more flexible to accommodate the development needs of low-income countries. The PRGF project team took the advice and completed the reform in 2010. In order to meet the increasing costs in production, trade and logistics, PRGF raised the standards and ceiling for concessional loans. The loan conditions are loosened and the interest rate is checked and adjusted every two years, reduced to zero at the end of 2016. Eligible countries with sound macroeconomic growth could receive "mixed" financial support, including non-concessional and concessional funds, from the IMF.

7.2.3 Poverty-Reduction Strategy Plan

Both the HIPC and PRGF are based on the PRSP, a country-level plan for economic, social and public administration over a three-year or longer period. It's prepared by the recipient government via extensive consultation with stakeholders such as the central and local governments, civil societies, individuals and international organizations. The World Bank and the IMF provide technical support in the setting of tracking indicators and related policy recommendations. The PRSP should provide the status quo of poverty, the main source of the poor people and assistance policies. In practice, there are Interim PRSP, Preparation Status Report, full-fledged PRSP and Annual Progress Report. As of 2016, 67 countries had submitted their respective PRSP to the World Bank and the IMF.

The PRSP is of particular importance for African countries. It initially served as the basis of the HIPC Initiative and is now the core policy document for recipient countries to negotiate with the IMF and the World Bank.

---

[3]Independent Evaluation Office of International Monetary Fund (2007).

The PRSP must meet three core requirements. First, it should be based on extensive public participation and national sovereignty, which is the core requirement. It must be based on extensive discussions in diversified forms, so as to demonstrate the independence and sovereignty of recipient countries in the formulation process. Second, the PRSP must reflect the country's priorities in poverty reduction and economic growth to achieve sustained growth in terms of macroeconomic indicators through structural reforms. On the premise of ensuring economic growth, PRGF is flexible and can be adjusted in line with the national conditions, but the IMF's approval is required. Third, to help recipient countries rationally design and implement PRGF programs, the IMF has laid stress on improving their governance capacity by focusing on assessing the impact of the government's public resource management capabilities and key macro policies on poverty and society. The World Bank is mainly responsible for providing technical guidance on the design of poverty-reduction policies, including monitoring and evaluation of poverty reduction effects, social issues and poverty-reduction project budgets.

7.2.4 OECD-DAC

The Organization for Economic Co-operation and Development (OECD) is an intergovernmental economic organization committed to addressing the economic, social and government management challenges that arise in globalization. Its Development Assistance Committee (DAC) is the traditional department dedicated to global poverty reduction, responsible for organizing, managing and supervising the implementation of official development assistance (ODA) in DAC member countries, with a focus on education, employment, trade and gender equality. At the same time, the OECD has been attracting growing importance to friendly cooperation with non-member countries to share knowledge and experience.

To assist in the achievement of the UN SDGs, the OECD has made some adjustments. In particular, the "Total Official Support for Sustainable Development" (TOSSD) is launched to enhance the transparency of ODA and evaluate and monitor the quality of ODA. To make up for the deficiencies of the ODA, TOSSD expands the framework for development financing to include traditional ODA, development funds from private institutions like Bill & Melinda Gates Foundation, and even broader sources of funding such as direct investment. The TOSSD concept and statistical approach are proposed by OECD-DAC to align with the SDGs, and to adjust its development assistance framework to South–South cooperation.

7.3 Challenges Facing Global Poverty Governance

7.3.1 Stubbornly Large Poor Population

The past few decades have seen remarkable progress in global poverty reduction. By the World Bank's reckoning based on the poverty line of USD 1.9 per day, the global incidence of poverty dropped from 44% in 1981 to 37.1% in 1990 before hitting 12.7% in 2012, while the poor population fell from 1.99 billion in 1981 to 1.958 billion in 1990 before reaching 902 million in 2012. East Asia has made outstanding achievements in eradicating extreme poverty, evidenced by the declining incidence of poverty from around 80% in 1981 to 7.2% in 2012, in which China played a decisive role. South Asia lagged slightly behind, with the incidence of poverty down from 58% in 1981 to 18.7% in 2012.

In sharp contrast, the incidence of poverty in Africa remained above 40% despite a steady stream of funds, materials, knowledge, experts, volunteers and other forms of assistance from former colonial powers, multilateral development agencies, and NGOs over the past few decades. From 1990 to 2012, both the incidence of poverty and the population in extreme poverty continued to decline around the world, except in the sub-Saharan Africa where the incidence of poverty was decreasing, but the incidence of extreme poverty approached 50% due to the excessively high growth rate of population (see Table 7.1).

Apart from the stubbornly high incidence of poverty, Africa performs poorly in terms of infrastructure, education, employment, social security and gender equality. When the country is backward on the whole, even the individuals and families who have shaken off poverty will find it difficult to sustain development and are highly likely to be reduced to poverty again by some financial crisis, natural disaster or disease.

Table 7.1 Poverty in the world and the sub-Saharan Africa

	Population (million)		Poor population (million)		Poverty headcount ratio[a] (%)	
	1990	2012	1990	2012	1990	2012
World	5,283	7,089	1,958	902	37.10	12.70
SSA	5,08.5	1,000.9	288.8	430.8	56.80	42.70

[a]Poverty headcount ratio at USD 1.90 a day (2011 PPP)
Source http://povertydata.worldbank.org/. Accessed on September 18, 2016

7.3.2 Failure in Delivering Structural Adjustment Dividends to the Poor

The Washington Consensus is the foundation of the World Bank, IMF and other international banks and financial institutions in dealing with development-oriented poverty-reduction issues, especially in the 1990s. They believe that economic growth is the premise of poverty reduction. In a poor country, only through economic growth can social capital and welfare trickle down to the poor people on the margins and allow them to share the dividends of economic growth. Therefore, the most fundamental purpose of the Washington Consensus is to establish a free and open market. Poor countries should learn from their rich counterparts to carry out structural reforms and establish a market economy system.

After 2005, the World Bank began to adopt a more conservative attitude towards the Washington Consensus. As indicated in the report titled "Economic Growth in the 1990s" by the World Bank,[4] it has been realized that the inequality and unsustainable problems brought by economic growth act much faster than the so-called trickle-down effect, and thus shifted its focus to human capital investment, inequality reduction and inclusive growth.

7.3.3 Limited Role of Good Governance

Another key influencer of global poverty governance is the change in the definition of poverty. Prior to the 1990s, the correlation between "governance" and "poverty reduction" was not obvious. Until the 1990s when the definition of poverty was expanded from "insufficient income" to include "deprivation of capabilities," the definition of poverty around the world has evolved from the single dimension of income to multiple dimensions concerning education, medical care, health and others. Accordingly, the mainstream concept in poverty reduction has developed from increasing income to a more "people-centered" strategy. During the same period, the World Bank and the IMF ended the strategy of structural adjustment in underdeveloped regions in pursuit for new poverty reduction strategies. In this context, the concept of "good governance" won the recognition of the world's main development institutions and gradually evolved into today's key poverty-reduction programs conducted by the Western countries in Africa.

What is governance? According to the UNDP, governance refers to the exercise of economic, political and administrative authority at all levels to manage a country's affairs. It comprises the mechanisms, processes and institutions, through which citizens and groups articulate their interests, exercise their legal rights, meet their obligations and mediate their differences. Good governance is, among other

---

[4]The World Bank. *Economic Growth in the 1990 s: Learning from a Decade of Reform.* World Bank Publications, Washington.

things, participatory, transparent and accountable. It is also effective and equitable. And it promotes the rule of law.[5]

In this context, the key words for good governance include participation, accountability, equality, rights, among others. The establishment of a democratic, transparent state ruled by law by virtue of the political system reform is the only way toward the fundamental driving force for development. Such good governance has gradually evolved into a prerequisite for developing countries to receive assistance. However, the empirical evidence concerning the establishment of good governance system for more than two decades showed that the state governance reform has a limited role in poverty reduction in Africa. The establishment of good governance didn't directly lead to poverty reduction in these least developed countries.[6] In other words, economic growth is a prerequisite for social development in these regions, and a blind copy of Western governance structure won't lead to poverty reduction through trickle-down effect envisioned by Western countries.

7.3.4 Declining Bilateral Aids

Problems also emerged in the bilateral poverty governance. The ODA from traditional DAC member states has continued to decline. Apart from the impact of financial crisis and domestic issues in economic development, another key reason is that years of ineffective aids has made developed countries reluctant to fulfill such "obligations." In many African countries, the per capita aid received is far outgrowing per capita income. Instead of doing any good, the aids turned out to be a burden for developed countries.[7] Such aid fatigue of the developed countries also became a major concern of the international community. At the Fourth High-Level Forum on Aid Effectiveness held in Busan, the Republic of Korea in 2011, the Busan Partnership for Effective Development Co-operation was endorsed: though controversial, it acknowledges the inefficiency of traditional development assistance and proposes to reform the ODA system to absorb a wider range of donors, especially the emerging economies, private sectors, civil societies, and social organizations.[8]

The debate on the effectiveness of aid has been ongoing for a long time without reaching a broad consensus in the world. Some scholars opined that the ODA advocated by the DAC member states over the past years had not been effective at all. For instance, Dambisa Moyo[9] pointed out that the Western countries' condescending aids for years, instead of improving the people's livelihood in Africa, inhibited the countries' sovereignty for development. African countries were deprived of the chances

[5]UNDP (1997).

[6]Kwon and Kim (2014).

[7]Easterly (2006).

[8]Zhong and Li (2013).

[9]Moyo (2010).

to develop independently in terms of public financial resources, government operations and industrial development, and even their national psychology and national culture were negatively affected. In this way, Africa became increasingly dependent on foreign aids. In response to such ineffective aids, the Africa must wean itself off aid, as if off the "drug addiction," so as to bring itself back on the path of independent development based on efficient utilization of resources, instead of entirely relying on foreign aids.

7.3.5 Dissimilation of Poverty-Reduction Projects

In Africa, the poverty-reduction projects of international organizations, sovereign states or international NGOs are almost close to perfect in design, but their design has never been faithfully translated into reality, and sometimes is even dissimilated.

Conditional and gifted assistance, instead of bringing the country onto the development track, has spawned rampant corruptions in African countries and ruined the possibility and opportunity for Africa's independent development.[10] Rampant corruption of African governments has not only led to a waste of the ODA, but more importantly, a serious harm to their own people. Due to the lack in the sense of security and rights, nearly one in five Africans paid bribes to government authorities to seek shelter or access to food, health, education, housing, and other basic needs. Such corruption not only severely hampers economic growth and social progress, but more importantly, leads to social exclusion.[11]

For quite a few countries, the PRSP is not merely an application or assessment report submitted to the World Bank and the IMF, but also a tool for presidential campaigns and party rivalry. The poverty-reduction strategies designed for political elections are not based on the national conditions, so cannot be effectively implemented and only end up in paperwork in most cases.

The developed countries' economic assistance to Africa may have failed, but their cultural interventions have exerted a profound impact. Having long engaged in the promotion of aids and governance concepts, they have infiltrated and influenced the African culture in an all-round way, making traditional African culture more fragmented and off the mainstream. In addition, due to the popularity of democratic governance in school education, the well-educated Africans tend to identify with overseas cultures, and their applications are more likely to be accepted by foreign universities and international institutions. These African elites, after finishing their overseas study, usually choose to stay, instead of going back to Africa. To worsen the brain-drain issue, Africa lacks effective policies to attract them back.

---

[10] Liu (2011).

[11] Milena Veselinovic (2016).

7.4 Summary

The United Nations, the IMF, the World Bank and the OECD-DAC are main institutions engaged in global poverty reduction. Generally speaking, international development agencies devise the poverty-reduction strategy in line with their own characteristics and areas of expertise. For instance, the poverty reduction of the World Bank and the IMF has centered on economic growth, while the WTO and the OECD have prioritized the aid for trade. With the deepening of globalization, independent operations of these development agencies can no longer satisfy the needs for current development of global poverty governance. The latest plight of global poverty reduction requires more daring and innovative development concepts, which presents opportunities for the emerging South–South cooperation led by China based on a win–win strategy.

The governance structure for global poverty reduction has been established and remained relatively firm. Developed countries (mainly bilateral aids) and multilateral aid institutions, based on democratic politics, economic and social development experience of developed countries, devised a variety of good plans for developing countries. Though controversial, these plans have contributed to the structure of global poverty governance.

To fulfill the 2030 SDGs in poverty reduction, the global poverty governance mechanism needs further improvement. The emerging economies' experience in development and poverty reduction which is independent from international development assistance, particularly China's poverty reduction model, deserves worldwide attention. This book draws a map of China's poverty governance at great length in the hope of providing valuable lessons for global poverty governance, and focuses on China's role in global poverty governance in this final chapter.

References

Easterly, W. (2006). *The white man's Burden: Why the West's efforts to Aid the rest have done so much Ill and so little good* (Hardcover). USA: Penguin Group.

Independent Evaluation Office of International Monetary Fund. (2007). An evaluation of the IMF and Aid to Sub-Saharan, Washington, D.C. http://www-ieo.imf.org/ieo/pages/CompletedEvaluation113.aspx.

Kwon, H-J., & Kim, E. (2014). Poverty reduction and good governance: Examining the rationale of the Millennium Development Goals. *Development and Change*, *45*(2), 353–375.

Li, X., Tang, L., & Wu, J. (2009). *International development assistance: Evolution, management and institutions* (pp. 18–43), Social Sciences Academic Press (China).

Liu, H. (2011). Rise from the ashes—Review on "Dead Aid". In D. Moyo (Ed.). *West Asia and Africa* (Vol. 7).

Loewe, M. (2014). Millennium plus or sustainable development goals: How to combine human development objectives with targets for global public goods? In *World outlook* (Vol. 4).

Moyo, D. (2010). *Dead aid: Why aid is not working and how there is a better way for Africa*. USA: Farrar, Straus and Giroux.

The World Bank. (2005). *Economic Growth in the 1990s: Learning from a decade of reform.* Washington: World Bank Publications.
UNDP. (1997). *Governance for sustainable human development.*
Veselinovic, M. (2016). Why corruption is holding Africa back, CNN News. http://edition.cnn.com/2015/12/24/africa/africa-corruption-transparency-international/index.html.
Zhong, L., & Li, X. (2013). The Busan partnership for effective development co-operation and its latest progress. *Journal of Guangxi University (Philosophy and Social Sciences), 2.*

The manufacturer's authorised representative in the EU is Springer Nature Customer Service Centre GmbH, Europaplatz 3, 69115 Heidelberg, Germany. If you have any concerns regarding our products, please contact ProductSafety@springernature.com

Printed and bound by CPI Group (UK) Ltd, Croydon, CR0 4YY
30/09/2026
02225574-0005